THE **MIRACLE** OF
REGENERATIVE
MEDICINE

"*The Miracle of Regenerative Medicine* is an inside job, a roadmap for readers who wish to get to the root cause of disease and take charge of their health. The science-based healing advice is especially helpful for brain, heart, and gut health. I highly recommend it. Read it and do it."

WILLIAM SEARS, M.D., COAUTHOR OF
THE DR. SEARS T5 WELLNESS PLAN

"We can direct and slow the aging of our bodies to be long-lived and in good health. Dr. Elisa Lottor clearly guides us to healthy longevity in her new book, *The Miracle of Regenerative Medicine*. She provides a comprehensive and completely useful guide for those wisely choosing to positively modulate their aging processes. Dr. Lottor tells us how to influence the evolution of our bodies and minds toward maximum health and consequent enjoyment of life. A must-read for anyone wanting to live better longer!

PRISCILLA SLAGLE, M.D., PSYCHIATRIST IN THE PRIVATE
PRACTICE OF NUTRITIONAL AND FUNCTIONAL MEDICINE &
PSYCHIATRY AND AUTHOR OF THE WAY UP FROM DOWN

"Dr. Lottor's book has arrived just in time for all of us aware of the huge transformation happening today in regenerative medicine! This book will become one of your most valuable resources and will not wander far from your bedside table. I have spent nine years in regenerative science research and Dr. Lottor has definitely given us the roadmap to the new life that awaits us. Excellent work!"

SUSAN B. SCHMIDT, M.L.S., RESEARCHER FOR
REGENERATIVE SCIENCES RESEARCH AND WRITER OF
THE NEWSLETTER *MEDICINE FOR A NEW ERA*

"A marvelous, simple-to-understand, and comprehensive book for people who want to stay young and live healthily. Dr. Lottor herself is a great example of self-care, vitality, and happiness."

CHIYAN WANG, A TAOIST LIGHT QIGONG LINEAGE
HOLDER (A 3,000-YEAR-OLD PRACTICE)
WITH 34 YEARS OF HEALING EXPERIENCE

THE **MIRACLE** OF

···

REGENERATIVE

···

MEDICINE

HOW TO NATURALLY
REVERSE THE AGING PROCESS

Elisa Lottor, Ph.D., H.M.D.

Healing Arts Press
Rochester, Vermont • Toronto, Canada

Healing Arts Press
One Park Street
Rochester, Vermont 05767
www.HealingArtsPress.com

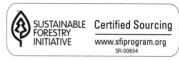

Text stock is SFI certified

Healing Arts Press is a division of Inner Traditions International

*Note to the reader: This book is intended as an informational guide. The remedies,
approaches, and techniques described herein are meant to supplement, and not to be a
substitute for, professional medical care or treatment. They should not be used to treat a
serious ailment without prior consultation with a qualified health care professional. Any
resemblance to actual persons living or dead or actual events is purely coincidental.*

Library of Congress Cataloging-in-Publication Data

Names: Lottor, Elisa, 1942–
Title: The miracle of regenerative medicine : how to naturally reverse the
    aging process / Elisa Lottor, Ph.D., HMD.
Description: Rochester, Vermont : Healing Arts Press, [2017] | Includes
    bibliographical references and index.
Identifiers: LCCN 2017026367 (print) | LCCN 2017018088 (e-book) |
    ISBN 9781620556030 (paperback) | ISBN 9781620556047 (e-book)
Subjects: LCSH: Aging—Prevention. | Regenerative medicine. | Nutrition. |
    Self-care, Health. | BISAC: HEALTH & FITNESS / Alternative Therapies. |
    SELF-HELP / Aging.
Classification: LCC RA776.75 (print) | LCC RA776.75 .L678 2017 (e-book) |
    DDC 613.2—dc23
LC record available at https://lccn.loc.gov/2017018088

Printed and bound in the United States by Lake Book Manufacturing, Inc.
The text stock is SFI certified. The Sustainable Forestry Initiative® program promotes
sustainable forest management.

10 9 8 7 6 5 4 3 2 1

Text design and layout by Priscilla Baker
This book was typeset in Garamond Premier Pro with Tide Sans, Avant Garde, Myriad
Pro, and Gill Sans used as display typefaces

To send correspondence to the author of this book, mail a first-class letter to the author
c/o Inner Traditions • Bear & Company, One Park Street, Rochester, VT 05767, and we
will forward the communication.

The Dalai Lama, when asked what surprised him most about humanity, answered, "Man, because he sacrifices his health in order to make money. Then he sacrifices money to recuperate his health. And then he is so anxious about the future that he does not enjoy the present; the result being that he does not live in the present or the future; he lives as if he is never going to die, and then dies having never really lived."

♪

This book is dedicated in memory of my mother, Rebecca Barocas Tacher, my husband, Michael, who has always been the wind beneath my wings, and my little girl, Resolina, who continues to be the love of my life.

You may think you met someone by accident, or that it was just a coincidence, but one day you will look back as I do and see how God used that person in an instrumental way to help you move closer to your divine destiny.

JOEL OSTEEN

This book could not have been written without the assistance of the following people who have gone above and beyond the call of duty to help, encourage, and support me throughout the process of writing this book: Bob Alonzi, Certified Advanced Rolfer; Ann Marie O'Farrell; and Chiyan Wang, Taoist Light Yoga.

I am truly grateful to Dr. David Y. Wong, Health Integration Center, and Dr. Julian Whitaker, the Whitaker Wellness Institute, who continue to teach and inspire me in ways they can't imagine.

I am also truly grateful to Oprah Winfrey and Dr. Mehmet Oz for dispensing state-of-the-art information on the health of the body, mind, and spirit to the widest audience possible; they truly embody this quote:

When you do things from your soul, you feel a river moving in you, a joy.

RUMI

CONTENTS

PART 3
The Search for a Solution

PART 4
Take Charge of Your Life

FOREWORD

JUDI GOLDSTONE, M.D.

Living a long and healthy life is much different today than it was in previous generations. It is actually possible, and a choice you can make. What does it take to get into top physical and mental shape and maintain it for a lifetime? What decisions can you make now to enjoy a long life of health, energy, enthusiasm, and feeling terrific? *The Miracle of Regenerative Medicine* by Dr. Elisa Lottor has all the answers and a game plan to put them into action as well. The fascinating, novel concepts in *The Miracle of Regenerative Medicine* are presented in such a compelling and practical manner that it is a must read for anyone wishing to be in control of his or her own destiny. Start now and take advantage of this remarkable book, which is on the forefront in the science, technology, and medicine of life extension, regeneration, and disease prevention.

Given the right circumstances, the body has the ability to heal and regenerate itself. It is possible to regain or improve health and vitality with aging. However, knowledge of what is currently available and/or is on the horizon in medicine, science, and technology is necessary in order to make proper choices for optimal health and well-being. Scientific advances to improve life-span and quality of life are being discovered continually but they can be difficult to find and integrate into a workable personal plan.

Dr. Lottor has been involved with the fastest growing and cutting-edge medical field of advanced preventive/regenerative/anti-aging medicine since its inception. All you have to do is read her book and utilize the strategies presented. She has done all the work by combining revelations from current scientific research and her forty years of clinical experience and patient feedback into this one powerful resource. *The Miracle of Regenerative Medicine* is the most comprehensive evaluation and explanation of existing advances and cutting-edge trends in disease detection, treatment, prevention, and reversal that I have read to date. I believe this is the only book necessary to read in order to gain the necessary knowledge and empower yourself to make wise choices for your future health and longevity.

Beside all the information presented, Dr. Lottor presents numerous scientifically validated tips and practical advice you can incorporate right now to prevent, reverse, and treat bodily degeneration. It is only with this incredible innovative information that you will be able to make informed, wise choices to regain, improve, and/or maintain your health and remain at your physical and mental peak for life.

My personal story, which is the story of a majority of my patients, illustrates why it is crucial to take charge of your health, learn as much as you can, and make the proper choices now. When I was in my midfifties, it seemed as though my body was rapidly deteriorating. I had no energy, was depressed, lost my enthusiasm for life, couldn't concentrate, and was barely able to work. I couldn't imagine that this was how life was supposed to be; was it all over at fifty? I didn't know where to go for help or even find information on what was happening. Several medical professionals told me it was just the natural aging process and there was nothing to do about it. Refusing to believe or accept this, I started a long, solo, and difficult learning process that lasted several years. What I discovered turned out to be life changing. Gradually, I was able to reverse these signs and symptoms of "aging" and return to optimal mental and physical functioning by incorporating a multimodality, holistic lifestyle approach, all of which is delineated in this book. If I, as a board certified, top internal medicine physician, had minimal knowledge of advanced, preventive, regenerative medicine, I imagine many people lack this information and could benefit greatly by learning about and incorporating the suggestions found in this book. Because of *The Miracle of Regenerative Medicine* you can be saved from the struggle many people experience with illness and aging. So, take advantage of this precious gift that will allow you to take control of your health and live a long, happy, and healthy life.

JUDI GOLDSTONE, M.D., is a board certified internal medicine physician. She is a long-standing member of the American Academy of Anti-Aging and Regenerative Medicine and the Obesity Medicine Association. Dr. Goldstone graduated at the top of her class from Mount Sinai School of Medicine in New York and has practiced weight loss and wellness medicine for the past fifteen years. She is a well-known expert in bioidentical hormone replacement therapy, nutraceautical usage, and nutrition. She practices at Southern California Center for Anti-Aging in Torrance, California.

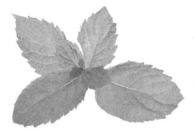

THE NEXT FRONTIER

Through the thicket of vines, a man and his party whip their machetes. The swords glimmer with the slashing motions, and the sunlight filters through the dense forest canopy. Sweat and the heavy air attract lazy swarms of mosquitos, which the men occasionally slap away before continuing forward. They are weary. They have traveled far, crossing oceans and trudging past the shores of the warm Atlantic coast.

They are searching restlessly, endlessly in these isles of Florida for a miraculous spring of water. Legend has it that this mysterious spring has the power to restore life, youth, and vitality to anyone who drinks of it. The captain has heard countless stories of its waters in his childhood; he has studied dusty tomes that claimed of its existence; and yet . . .

The man wipes his forehead and leans back on a tree, feeling the rough bark against his drenched shirt. He watches the men continue their work. In this very moment, he can only imagine how refreshing it would feel to drink deeply from the clear waters. To splash and laugh in the waves, like a child. To float weightlessly on his back, freed of every burden. To wash away the weariness settled deep inside his bones. No, he mustn't only imagine. Juan Ponce de León must obtain, once and for all, the wondrous powers of the Fountain of Youth.

Juan Ponce de León may be considered the patron saint of the Fountain of Youth, but the sixteenth-century explorer wasn't the only one to seek the powers of rejuvenation. Tales of the fountain resonate throughout history and geography over the span of thousands of years. The Greek historian Herodotus—widely regarded as the Father of History—describes his encounter with the miraculous water near the lands of Egypt, in the fifth century BCE. The water reputedly granted longevity, as well as stature and good looks to the inhabitants of Macrobia. And according to the legends of the East, Alexander the Great journeyed through the Lands of Darkness—the impenetrable forest that doomed its inhabitants to eternal wandering—to seek the coveted Water of Life. Even the Bible features its own fountain of healing in the Pool of Bethesda. According to the fifth chapter of the Gospel of John, an angel would descend to stir the miraculous pools, bestowing complete restoration to the first who entered its waters.

These texts characterize the Fountain of Youth as an element of myth, legend, and even miracle. Indeed, the fountain seems to inhabit a space beyond our everyday lives, in an atmosphere of fantasy and faith. If we were to trace the fountain back to its roots, we would not be surprised to see it emerge from the depths of human imagination, a desperate fantasy to cope with the ever-present decay of the body. But although eternal youth and everlasting life may be entirely fictional, the coming chapters will demonstrate that biological rejuvenation lies perfectly within our reach. Whether we desire to maintain our health, or long for the energy and focus of our youth, regenerative medicine promotes healthy, holistic, and natural solutions that will work to reverse the passage of time.

Biological rejuvenation lies perfectly within our reach.

Before we look for a solution, we must first evaluate the problem: growing old. From a scientific standpoint, aging begins at birth. It is the continuing process of development and degeneration, in body and in mind. Time, gravity, environment, stress—each of these works to damage the body and propel us steadily toward death. However, the body doesn't passively sit and allow its own demise: from cuts and bruises to colds and infections, the body heals and protects itself through cell regeneration and the immune system.

Now, let's extend this natural healing process to a broader medical theory: if the body naturally heals and regenerates by itself, it may even be able to counteract the minute but persistent daily wear that our cells face over time. By renewing and replacing old cells, our bodies could effectively turn back the biological clock—under the right circumstances. That's where we come in: when we pay close attention to our bodies' language and provide ourselves with the best-known resources, our bodies will undoubtedly reach their full regenerative potential.

> **Our bodies could turn back the biological clock—under the right circumstances.**

Contrary to popular belief, regenerative medicine is not an anti-aging effort. It does not aim to slow or stop the aging process. Instead, regenerative medicine aims to *reverse* the process by improving the efficiency of our biochemistry and cell functions, thereby promoting self-healing and recovery. Consider it parallel to the human mental capacity: though we each have our own peak levels of brain activity and function, we don't always achieve it. But if we were to fully understand the brain and the way memory, logic, and analysis work, we could utilize *more* of our brain power, more effectively. Similarly, when we begin to understand our bodies intimately and personally, we increase our bodily capacity for healing and recovery, as well as rejuvenation.

> **Regenerative medicine improves the quality of our lives through years of freedom and happiness.**

Regenerative medicine does not focus on the superficial: it doesn't target appearances, like plastic surgery, or external symptoms, like pharmaceutical drugs. It doesn't aim only to increase the *number* of years we gain, because what is the use of a longer life without personal empowerment and independence? Instead, regenerative medicine improves the *quality* of the life we live, and gives us more years of freedom and happiness.

We as a society are entering a paradigm shift: as patients grow more familiar with alternative and complementary medicine, doctors are beginning to realize that traditional modes of medicine often neglect individual care. Whereas traditional medicine aims to *combat the disease,* regenerative medicine aims to *treat the patient* through the implementation of comprehensive lifestyle changes.

Regenerative medicine uses scientific research as a tool to better understand the origin of our strengths and our struggles—the body. Contrary to traditional medicine, regenerative medicine does not wait for the disease to occur. Rather, it takes preventive measures by confronting disease at its very roots. It always pursues a permanent solution through the use of natural compounds such as vitamins, minerals, nutraceuticals, herbs, bioidentical hormones, and the unobtrusive practice of energy medicine.

Regenerative medicine lies on the cutting-edge frontier of scientific research. As a relatively new scientific and medical discipline, it pays particular attention to harnessing the power of stem cells as well as the body's natural regenerative capacity to restore function to damaged cells, tissues, and organs. You may have heard of this already—scientists are developing stem cells into specific cell types so as to be able to repair, replace, or even *grow* new functioning organs.

In 2011, for example, nineteen-year-old marine Isaias Hernandez lost his right leg to a mortar in Afghanistan. He took such severe muscle damage up his thigh that ordinarily he would have had to have it amputated. However, the U.S. military invested $70 million in an experimental regenerative procedure that extracted a growth hormone from pig bladders to inject into his leg. These hormones stimulated his remaining muscle matter to regenerate, and eventually, after sufficient care and recovery, Hernandez found his leg—and his life—fully restored.

Regenerative medicine aims to heal the body from within.

More recently, in April 2013, a newborn baby, born without a trachea (windpipe) was implanted with a bioengineered organ in a hospital in Illinois. Dr. Paolo Macchinari led the procedure, taking stem cells from the baby's own bone marrow and artificially incubating the organ until it was ready to be implanted. This gave her a new chance at life. She survives to this very day, and though she may need replacement surgeries as her body continues to grow, the fact that she has the capacity to grow in the first place is nothing short of miraculous. Developments like these represent huge steps of progress in regenerative medicine. Because, in the end, regenerative medicine does not incorporate artificial products that may cause unforeseen bodily rejections or consequences. It aims to heal the body from within.

Imagine a future without painful backs and knees—a future in which our own bodies will repair the worn-out joints that cause arthritis and inflammation. Imagine a future without the endless delay for an organ donor, because we will be able to grow our own skin, our own bones, our own livers and kidneys and hearts. Imagine a wellspring of healing for blindness, deafness, and even paralysis. Open your eyes: the future is here.

Growing older is a natural process, but *feeling* old is entirely optional. Our medical tool kit has never been so vast, versatile, and readily available. Our generation can not only experience *longer* life-spans, but also enjoy vitality, health, and wellness far into our autumn years. We work hard throughout our lives: pursuing careers, raising kids, maintaining an entire household. Don't we deserve something better as we age, when we have the leisure to enjoy life with those we love?

What's stopping us?

> *The secret to change is to focus all your energy not into fighting the old, but on building the new.*
>
> SOCRATES

PART 1

What's the Matter?

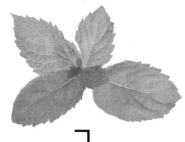

1
INFLAMMATION
The Root of Disease

A good doctor endeavors to help the body repair itself, to awaken the healer within.

J. E. BLOCK, M.D.

Barbara sat in her doctor's office while she rattled off a litany of complaints. She had arthritis in her hands and knees, and they ached all the time, her dentist just told her she had gingivitis, and now, she had just been diagnosed with gastritis. She was only forty-five. She wanted to know what was going on. You might be thinking, she's so young to have so many health problems, but people a lot younger have even more serious and chronic problems. "My body seems to be falling apart," she said. If truth be told, she looked a lot older than forty-five. Her diet and lifestyle were finally catching up, even before she reached menopause.

> **Your body's ability to heal is greater than anyone has permitted you to believe.**

Of course, her doctor prescribed pain pills for her and told her to take Aleve, but he failed to inform her what the underlying factor contributing to all her health problems was: it was inflammation. Words that end in *itis* mean inflammation, like laryngitis, the inflammation of the larynx, or conjunctivitis, the inflammation of the membrane that covers the eye (known as conjunctiva). She had arthritis, the inflammation of the joints; gingivitis, the inflammation of the gums; and gastritis, the inflammation of the stomach. Her body was telling her that something was very wrong.

> **If you can put out the fire of inflammation, many,**
> **if not most, health problems would dissipate.**

Chronic inflammation is a newly identified cause of many health problems from diabetes to heart disease, which is the number one killer in Western countries. In fact, if you can put out the fire of inflammation that is going on in the body, many, if not most, health problems would dissipate. If this is the case, then why are we living with so many diseases in our lives?

When Barbara called to make an appointment, I asked her to bring in a food journal of everything she had consumed for the past week and write down the type and duration of exercise and how many hours she slept, and the quality of her sleep. When she came for her first visit, I could tell by the extra weight she carried and where she carried it (around her waist), that she not only did not exercise, but also ate a diet of refined foods, sodas, and a little too much alcohol. She said, "I have a couple of glasses of wine when I come home to unwind, and sometimes I drink more than I know is good for me." This was evident from her blotchy complexion, dull hair with split ends, and bloodshot eyes. I could also tell that she was suffering from adrenal exhaustion because of the dark circles under her eyes. I later found out that she was a single mother and was working full time while having to cook, clean, and take care of her children. It was obviously taking its toll. Additionally, she was getting about six hours of sleep per night.

> **Inflammation is the mother of all diseases.**

After reading her food and exercise journal, I was not surprised to find out that my suspicion was right. She did not exercise and consumed a diet of sugar and refined foods. I explained to her that both her diet and sedentary lifestyle, along with a lack of sufficient sleep and increased stress were causing all her health issues. She was not a happy camper. I presented several suggestions that could help quell her inflammation and improve her overall health. These included changing her diet, finding stress-management techniques other than alcohol, and getting a half hour of exercise on a daily basis. Also, I encouraged her to get enough sleep and take anti-inflammatory supplements. The prevalence of drinking in women has increased incrementally with their responsibilities of having to "do it all." Had she continued with her current lifestyle, she would not only be shortening her life-span, but she would also be creating the perfect storm for chronic disease.

Scientists have searched for and recently found out why some people live to be over one hundred, while being physically active, happy, and healthy. A team of experts in Tokyo researched which processes in the body may be responsible for not only successful aging but also for longevity. They have identified the common denominator, and that is inflammation. In this chapter, we will learn to not only identify the signs of chronic inflammation, but also what to do to keep it at bay.

Professor Thomas von Zglinicki from Newcastle University Institute for Ageing in the United Kingdom found that, "Centenarians and super-centenarians seem to age slower and they can ward off disease much longer than the general population."

> ### The level of inflammation predicts successful aging.

Inflammation increases with age, but those people who were successful in keeping inflammation under control invariably maintained good cognition, independence, and had extended years.

This study showed for the first time that the level of inflammation predicts successful aging. It is hoped that this understanding of extreme longevity can translate to the general population, helping them achieve an extended healthy life-span. Dr. Yasumichi Arai, Head of Tokyo Oldest Old Survey on Total Health said, "Our results suggest that mitigating chronic inflammation might help people to age more slowly."

Severe inflammation is an aspect of many aging-related diseases and the lifelong accumulation of molecular damage resulting from chronic inflammation has been suggested as a major contributor to the process of aging.

WHAT IS INFLAMMATION?

The concept of inflammation is probably one of the most exciting revelations to come to light in recent years because it points to the common denominator behind practically every disease.

What most health care practitioners neglect to inform you is that you can reduce inflammation in your body, thereby eliminating one of the major causes of disease and premature aging. According to the Centers for Disease Control, seven out of every ten deaths are attributed to cancer, heart disease, or diabetes. What do these all have in common? They are all linked to inflammation!

But what exactly is inflammation? We all have heard the term *inflammation* before, but we don't know exactly what it is and how big an effect it can have on our lives. At some point, we have all encountered inflammation. If you've sprained an ankle or bumped your head, you may have noticed swelling at the point where the injury happened. This is inflammation. It is the body's way of telling us that there is something wrong and that it is protecting itself from further damage by essentially padding the affected area. Acute inflammation also helps in the healing process by removing dead cells and helping in the regeneration of new cells.

However, there is a huge difference between acute and chronic inflammation. When inflammation becomes chronic, it is no longer a healthy immune response for healing the body; instead it becomes the root cause of a disease. Practically every chronic disease has inflammation as the underlying cause. Many common everyday health issues experienced by people are the result of chronic inflammation. A well-known form of inflammation is arthritis. "My arthritis is acting up" and "Arthritis just comes with age," can commonly be heard from the general population. You may think of this as an old people's ailment, but even younger people are showing symptoms of this inflammation much earlier in life than normal.

You might be wondering what you can do to treat or prevent such incidents from occurring. What if you could change the course of inflammation by simply making a few changes to your lifestyle? Well, you can! We are going to take a look at some small ways that can yield big results. But first let's talk about what causes inflammation.

THE CAUSES OF INFLAMMATION

How can we alleviate inflammation now that we know what it is? Knowing where inflammation comes from can help you to understand some simple and achievable ways to rid your body of this painful and possibly crippling condition.

When it comes to your health, ignorance is not bliss.

Most of our health problems are in one way or another attributed to inflammation. For example, due to the fact that they end with *-itis,* we know that arthritis, bursitis, diverticulitis, and other *-itis* problems connect directly to inflammation. But did you also know that other diseases, such as heart disease and cancers, can directly result from inflammation? Knowing this, we need to find the causes of inflammation so that we can stop chronic health problems before they begin. So, what causes inflammation and why do we need to know about it?

Here are some factors that can contribute to chronic inflammation:

- Being obese or overweight: having a waist size of over 35 inches if you're a woman, and over 40 inches if you're a man
- Eating a poor diet, high in sugar (even fructose) and refined carbohydrates and unhealthy oils
- A genetic predisposition or history of heart disease
- Prediabetes or diabetes
- A sedentary lifestyle, sitting too much
- Smoking tobacco, drinking too much alcohol (more than 4 oz. per day)
- Having a chronic infection or autoimmune disease
- Chronic stress

Inflammation has direct links to our diet and lifestyle. As we look at Barbara's situation mentioned in the introduction, we notice that much of the inflammation relates to how she lives her life. She eats processed foods that contain large amounts of sugars, does not pursue regular physical activity, and has chronic, unremitting stress as well as lack of sufficient sleep. Breaking down her situation, we can see many causes of inflammation before we dig even deeper.

Let's take a look at some of the common factors that lead to inflammation that we can take control of right now.

Diet

When it comes down to it, the standard Western diet is largely responsible for inflammation. One hundred years ago, you wouldn't hear half the health complaints that we hear of today. In fact, even thirty years ago, when I began my practice, I never encountered patients with so many chronic diseases. What is one of the key differences between how they lived then and how we live now? People ate healthier and they got regular physical activity.

The standard Western diet is largely responsible for inflammation.

The story of Dr. Terry Wahls has some fascinating ties to how a diet can help, if not cure, illness. She was diagnosed with multiple sclerosis and was essentially crippled. While she followed the advice and treatments that were common to MS, she was still feeling its crippling effects. One day, she decided that she was going to put her research to the test. If she could change her diet to support her mitochondria and myelin sheaths, she felt she could change the course of her disease.

By taking on a paleo, whole-foods diet, she was able to reverse the effects of the disease and actually cure it. How can this be? She basically eliminated all of the foods that are linked to inflammation! The processed and refined foods that are common in the Western diet were purged from her diet, and she was able to reverse the effects of a crippling disease!

This goes to show that diet can play a huge role in how our bodies react to disease. If we can support our health by eliminating foods that can cause disease, we might actually be able to cure and prevent some of the most disabling diseases.

In the next chapter, I am going to go more into depth about the elements of our modern diet, but for now, I want to emphasize that what we eat is a common factor linked to inflammation. By eating refined and processed foods and foods that are high in sugar, we are not giving our bodies the nutrients that they need for growth, repair, and regeneration.

By making a few changes to our diet, we can make a huge change to our overall health. Later on in this chapter, I will present a few suggestions on how you can change your diet in small ways in order to avoid chronic inflammation.

Lifestyle

Another key factor in chronic inflammation is our modern lifestyle. Instead of walking, we drive places. In Southern California where I live, people often joke that they drive to their mailboxes. The effort it takes to do tasks today is much less than it was before technology came around. People were used to moving before gadgets that promoted ease came along.

Just because we have made our lives easier doesn't give us an excuse to stop moving. By finding opportunities to move and be active, we are using the calories our diet provides and allowing our joints to move more efficiently, controlling cortisol and other inflammatory processes in the body.

Inactivity, combined with a diet high in processed foods can lead to weight gain and inflammation. In fact, obesity is a problem we are now seeing even in children. A new term has been coined called *diabesity* to refer to a metabolic dysfunction that involves obesity and diabetes. At the beginning of this chapter, one of my main recommendations for Barbara was to get thirty minutes of activity in a day. This doesn't mean going to the gym and sweating it out on a treadmill. You can simply take a walk and enjoy nature!

Mind-Set

Along with diet and lifestyle, many people have adopted the mind-set that certain diseases are just a part of aging. This is simply not true. However, by thinking this, they live their lives expecting to have arthritis and other health problems. I am seeing more people now than ever before with several autoimmune diseases like fibromyalgia, Hashimoto's thyroiditis, and cancer.

Getting older does not mean you have to succumb to illness and disease. It is not necessarily a natural part of aging, even though the prevailing mentality is that it is. Also, not all old people are confined to walkers, canes, and wheelchairs. Most importantly, they don't take handfuls of prescription medication on a daily basis.

Recently, I watched a video on the internet about the world's oldest gymnast. She was ninety years old, and she had the flexibility of a teenager! She didn't let the standards of old age determine how she aged. When asked what her secret was, she stated that she ate right and exercised frequently. She didn't take supplements or other things to boost her health. She simply led a healthy lifestyle.

> *When you change the way you look at things, the things you look at change.*
>
> Wayne Dyer

Stress

Stress has a huge effect on our bodies in various ways. I have noted that many women use alcohol as a stress-reducing elixir. I have given lectures at women's groups and noted that women were drinking wine at 10:30 in the morning. When I questioned this, the answer I got is, "Wine is good for you."

One of my patients said, "When I used to stress out, I would make my way to the kitchen. Food was a comfort to me, and when I felt like my nerves were shot, I ate ice cream straight from the carton standing up by the sink, sometimes consuming the whole container."

One patient told me that her husband had brought home a cake for the company they were expecting that night. Well, she was so stressed out that she ended up eating the whole cake and had to make a quick run to the bakery to replace it, so her husband wouldn't know. Although the food tasted great and temporarily eased her nerves, it was highly processed and full of sugar. These are two of the main factors that can lead to inflammation.

> **Cortisol is the driver of inflammation.**

Additionally, when we are stressed out or don't get enough sleep, the body secretes more cortisol, which is the driver of inflammation. Knowing this, it becomes paramount that we learn how to handle stress. Diet and exercise are two ways, but in the subsequent chapters, we will go into detail about supplements, specific exercises, amounts of sleep, and ways to change our mindset that will change how we handle stress.

If I have to point to the worst dietary culprit, I would have to cite sugar. People are consuming 128 pounds of sugar a year. When sugar enters the body it releases inflammatory toxins that result in different types of inflammation. The sugar causes something known as glycation, which turns proteins into toxins. These hybrid proteins are called AGEs (Advanced Glycation End Products).

By eliminating or limiting our sugar intake, we can prevent these AGEs from forming in our bodies. Learning to substitute refined sugar with natural alternatives can make a huge difference in the ways in which we enjoy our foods.

Understanding the processes in our bodies that can result in inflammation will make us think twice the next time we want to dive into a sugary dessert!

KNOWING IF YOU HAVE CHRONIC INFLAMMATION

While inflammation can be a normal and healthy reaction to injury or infection, chronic inflammation can often be symptomless until you lose function in a particular part of your body. Knowing if you have chronic inflammation can help save your body from further damage.

The C-reactive protein blood test is one of a few medical tests that can be used to determine if there is a risk of chronic inflammation in the body. It is a blood test that can detect the proteins that can lead to inflammation. Another medical test that can help detect inflammation in the body is the ESR (erythrocyte sedimentation rate), which uses a fasting blood sugar test to determine the amount of insulin in your blood and risks for inflammation. The presence of excess insulin can indicate the presence of inflammation.

Even if you show few or no symptoms of inflammation, I would still like to encourage you to take steps to prevent it from occurring in the future. Preventing and detecting chronic inflammation early on can help prevent severe damage to your body.

Ron made an appointment with me at his doctor's suggestion after his C-reactive protein results were high. He wanted to know not only what that means, but also how he could lower his score. He wasn't totally convinced that there was a problem since he had no symptoms. I made the suggestions that are described in this chapter about cleaning up his diet and taking anti-inflammatory supplements, but he wasn't quite convinced and decided since he had no symptoms, why make changes. He tried to take aspirin that his doctor had recommended but it bothered his stomach.

A year later Ron ended up in the emergency room with a mild stroke (TIA). This time when he came for his appointment again, at his doctor's suggestion, he not only took notes, but brought in a tape recorder. He said, "I guess I should have taken your suggestions more seriously. I had no idea that inflammation was such a big deal."

HOW TO TREAT INFLAMMATION

Having chronic as opposed to acute inflammation is a sign that you need to make changes to your lifestyle. We can begin by eliminating sugar and moderating alcohol. Also, we can start eating a whole-foods, preferably home-cooked, diet with seasonal and locally grown foods and remove all processed foods from the diet.

We can begin a practice of meditation, yoga, t'ai chi, or qigong to control stress. Supplements can provide your body the necessary nutrients if you cannot get them in your diet. Some supplements that can help relieve inflammation include:

- A vitamin D supplement may be necessary if you do not get a lot of natural sunlight.

- Ginger offers anti-inflammatory benefits while also acting as a pain reliever and stomach soother, added as tea or a condiment on a daily basis.
- Bromelain is an enzyme that is found in pineapples that eases inflammation. You can take it as a supplement or eat fresh pineapple.
- Boswellia is an herb that contains active anti-inflammatory ingredients, referred to as boswellic acids, that have been proven to significantly reduce inflammation.
- Resveratrol is an antioxidant found in certain grapes, vegetables, and cocoa and is known to promote the look of youth. It keeps your body from forming sphingosine kinase and phospholipase D, which are known to trigger inflammation.
- Fish or krill oil is also a powerful anti-inflammatory containing omega-3 fatty acids and DHA.
- Turmeric, or curcumin, can often produce dramatic results.

Inflammation can be a silent killer.

Alongside taking supplements, some changes to your lifestyle like getting more exercise, quitting smoking, and finding healthier ways to handle high stress levels, other than alcohol, will help to keep inflammation in check.

Here are some ways chronic inflammation can be a silent killer:

- It can harm your gut.
- It can harm your joints.
- It's linked to heart disease.
- It's linked to a higher risk of cancer.
- It has recently been implicated in Alzheimer's disease.
- It can damage your gums.
- It can make weight loss more difficult.
- It can damage your bones.
- It can affect your skin.

In the next chapter, we will find out how people are living longer and healthier lives all over the world, unencumbered by pain and many of the afflictions we have come to associate with aging. We are going to read about these people in depth to find out their secret. It may also be fascinating to realize that these people don't have to take pain medications, cholesterol medication, high blood pressure medication, or use walkers or canes, hearing aids, or even glasses, but they can still move around as easily as someone half their age. Also, they are basically unencumbered with the ailments we have come to associate with aging; you may wonder what makes them so healthy.

But first let's take a look at some of the common foods that will help you to treat and prevent inflammation.

Anti-inflammatory foods include:

Fermented foods and beverages like yogurt, kimchi, sauerkraut, lebne, and kefir

Saturated fat-finding foods that are rich in omega-3 fatty acids rather than omega-6 fatty acids can drastically reduce inflammation and inflammatory symptoms in the body—try eating more fish, nuts, and seeds

Turkey: the chemical tryptophan, known for making us sleepy after a turkey dinner, also helps boost serotonin in your system, combating depression; selenium is another antidepressant found in turkey and it also has anti-inflammatory qualities

Dark chocolate: the chemicals in dark chocolate can help reduce pro-inflammatory C-reactive protein—enjoy a small cube of 70 percent dark chocolate daily to help reduce inflammation

Green tea: this beverage can help ease your stress while doubling as an anti-inflammatory

Legumes like beans and chickpeas: chickpeas contain tryptophan, folate, and vitamin B_6, all of which have great anti-inflammatory properties

A diet that includes many anti-inflammatory foods will help the existing inflammation to diminish and prevent new occurrences of inflammation. Along with foods that prevent inflammation, there is a list of foods that you should avoid in order to keep inflammation at bay.

Foods that are known to cause inflammation include:

Sugars: excessive use of sugars can result not only in inflammation, but also diseases such as diabetes, obesity, Alzheimer's disease, heart disease, and tooth decay. There are natural sugar alternatives such as stevia that will still give you the benefit of having the sweet taste without the inflammation!

Cooking oils: common cooking oils used in kitchens today are high in omega-6 fatty acids rather than omega-3 fatty acids. Omega-6 acids result in instances of inflammation and discomfort, while omega-3 acids are recommended to ease inflammation. Instead of using unhealthy vegetable oils for cooking, try using butter or olive oil or coconut oil. They are high in omega-3s!

Red and processed meats: these meats include a molecule that initiates an immune response in our bodies that may cause inflammation. Since our bodies cannot process this molecule, it is best to avoid it. Instead, try eating more fish and poultry. Also, if choosing to eat red meat, make sure that it is from grass-fed animals and is the leanest cut available.

Alcohol: high levels of alcohol consumption contribute to inflammation and possibly cancer. Try limiting your alcohol consumption to one drink, or four ounces a day, and fill the void with green tea or water.

Refined grains: these grains are processed until they lack all the nutrients and fiber that we look for in grains. By eating too many refined grains, we are filling ourselves with empty calories. Instead of consuming these, try eating foods made from whole grains. Take a closer look at labels when buying bread and cereals to make sure that your grains are truly whole grains!

Food with artificial additives and preservatives: these are common alternatives to sweeteners that we use today. Artificial additives and preservatives are only found in boxed foods. In order to avoid these, try making sure that you eat fresh food or that the food you do eat is sweetened naturally.

All of these foods contain agents that result in inflammation. While it may be impossible to avoid eating some of these completely, at least try to drastically reduce your consumption of these particular foods. Try to substitute these foods with better choices that will decrease inflammation.

BENEFITS OF EATING AN ANTI-INFLAMMATORY DIET

If you quell the fire of inflammation, not only will you prevent chronic disease that brings on more stress and medication, but you also allow your body to focus its energy on repairing itself. Using methods to alleviate and prevent inflammation can help you begin to live a healthier and more fulfilling life.

By eating an anti-inflammatory diet, you will see many benefits to your health including:

Increased energy, improved mood: having a better mindset will help you to cope with stresses more productively and view your lifestyle and diet in a more positive light

Better health: better elimination, improved sleep, and so forth will result in a dissipation of some chronic health problems

Improved skin (begins to glow): when your body rids itself of the toxins that cause inflammation, your skin will improve and glow

Healthier hair: eating a healthier diet will give your hair the nutrients it needs in order to promote a lustrous and full head of healthy hair

Improved blood pressure and cholesterol levels: giving your body what it needs will improve the function of your circulatory system and the cholesterol in your blood

Health is the new wealth.

A whole-foods diet has some wonderful benefits to your health and well-being. Not only will you look and feel better but you will create the appropriate terrain from which your body can begin the process of repair and regeneration.

POINTS TO REMEMBER

Chronic inflammation is often undetectable until it causes larger problems. Knowing that inflammation has a direct link to disease makes it worth focusing on changing our lives to prevent it. Not only can inflammation affect your inner health, it can also affect your physical appearance. To start making changes to your life you can:

- Eliminate or cut back on foods known to cause inflammation
- Get at least thirty minutes of exercise on a daily basis
- Substitute foods that will promote your body's healing processes
- Try substituting alcoholic beverages with water or green tea
- Find alternatives to stress relief rather than eating, or alcohol
- Improve your mind-set and change your common misconceptions of diet and disease
- Get enough good quality sleep
- Take anti-inflammatory supplements

Since inflammation is a huge factor in disease, finding ways to treat and prevent it can help boost your quality of life. I encourage you to try to find alternatives to the foods that you currently eat and make changes to your activity levels. Pay attention to what food you are buying and how you prepare it. All of these factors can make a huge difference in your feelings of health and well-being.

One might naturally wonder why I didn't write a book on inflammation alone, as it seems to be at the root of every disease. Well it's because inflammation is just the tip of the iceberg, just as pain is a symptom of something more. When the body engages in an inflammatory response it cannot mobilize its ability to heal and regenerate.

In subsequent chapters, we will learn about the elements that promote healing and regeneration. We will begin to understand where true health really comes from—and what you need to do to encourage it. You will learn how to plant the seeds of regeneration in the fertile soil of infinite possibilities.

REFERENCES FOR CHAPTER 1

Axe, Josh. "10 Anti-Inflammatory & Disease-Fighting Foods." *MindBodyGreen,* September 19, 2015. www.mindbodygreen.com/0-21664/10-anti -inflammatory-disease-fighting-foods.html (accessed April 29, 2017).

Benson, Jonathan. "Reduce Widespread Inflammation in Your Body with These Foods." *Natural News,* February 1, 2013. www.naturalnews.com/038915 _inflammation_foods_healing.html (accessed April 29, 2017).

Black, Jessica. "Prevent Illness with the Anti-Inflammatory Diet." *Mother Earth Living,* May/June 2015. www.motherearthliving.com/food-and-recipes/food -for-health/anti-inflammatory-diet-zmoz15mjzhou.aspx (accessed April 29, 2017).

Francis, Raymond. "Inflammation: A Common Denominator of Disease." *Arizona Center for Advanced Medicine,* June 26, 2013. www.arizonaadvancedmedicine .com/Articles/2013/June/Inflammation-A-Common-Denominator-of -Disease.aspx (accessed April 29, 2017).

Get Holistic Health. "Top 10 Inflammatory Foods to Avoid Like the Plague." July 12, 2013. www.getholistichealth.com/40185/top-10-inflammatory -foods-to-avoid-like-the-plague/ (accessed April 29, 2017).

Goldstein, Michelle. "Carbon Dioxide 'Pollutant' Myth Debunked: Eating for Happiness." *Natural News,* December 13, 2013. www.naturalnews .com/043226_happiness_organic_diet_processed_foods.html (accessed April 29, 2017).

Kahn, Joel. "Don't Overthink Your Diet, Just Eat More Plants: A Cardiologist Explains." *MindBodyGreen,* October 2, 2013. www.mindbodygreen.com /0-11149/dont-overthink-your-diet-just-eat-more-plants-a-cardiologist -explains.html (accessed April 29, 2017).

Marquis, David. "How Inflammation Affects Every Aspect of Your Health." *Mercola,* March 7, 2013. http://articles.mercola.com/sites/articles /archive/2013/03/07/inflammation-triggers-disease-symptoms.aspx (accessed April 29, 2017).

Nelson, Jennifer. "Is Inflammation the Root of All Health Evil?" *Mother Nature Network,* February 25, 2013. www.mnn.com/health/fitness-well-being /stories/is-inflammation-the-root-of-all-health-evil (accessed April 29, 2017).

Newcastle University. "Inflammation, Not Telomere Length, Predicts Healthy Longevity of Centenarians." *Medical Press,* April 5, 2015. http://medicalxpress

.com/news/2015-08-inflammation-telomere-length-healthy-longevity.html (accessed April 29, 2017).

Shemek, Lori. "9 Foods to Fight Inflammation and Boost Your Mood." *MindBodyGreen,* July 16, 2015. www.mindbodygreen.com/0-20729/9 -foods-to-fight-inflammation-boost-your-mood.html (accessed April 29, 2017).

WorldHealth.net. "Anti-Inflammation for Anti-Aging," September 25, 2015. Updated June 30, 2016. www.worldhealth.net/news/anti-inflammation -anti-aging/ (accessed April 29, 2017).

2
FOOD IS THE
BEST MEDICINE

It is health that is the real wealth, not pieces of gold and silver.

MAHATMA GANDHI

At Dave's 100th birthday party, everyone wanted to know to what he attributed his longevity. He spoke of how he grew up in Turkey in a very large, poor family. His mother would make the bread, they ate what fish they caught in the ocean, and had bread and olive oil or cheese for breakfast and lunch, and dinner was vegetable soup. He was eating the traditional diet of his region.

Whenever I hear of a centenarian or supercentenarian, I too always want to know what the "secret" is that contributes to his or her long life. Instead of asking each individual, we went directly to where the most long-lived people in the world were and found out that their diet was a big factor contributing to their longevity. We will take you on a journey to examine what they ate in the "Traditional Diet."

Even though it might be difficult to eat like Dave did growing up, we can still take measures to make our diets more like Dave's. We want to live a long and healthy life, so why not use those who are enjoying that life as our examples?

Food has a lot to do with our overall well-being.

Are you as intrigued as I am with long-lived people and what changes you can make to improve your health and vitality? You perhaps not only want to increase your life-span, but the quality of your older years as well. After all, we don't just want increased years, we want quality: we want to be active, vital, and healthy.

Food has a lot to do with our overall well-being. I want to encourage you to take a look at the ways that centenarians all over the world eat, going beyond the Mediterranean diet, and see if you can make some changes based on the research of these "time-proven" ways of eating.

SECRETS TO LONGEVITY

Every human being is the author of his own health and disease.

THE BUDDHA

In many Westernized countries like the United States, there are many people suffering from diseases due to inactive lifestyle and poor dietary choices. As consumers, we are constantly being bombarded with enticement for buying unhealthy foods.

It doesn't have to be this way. Making the necessary changes now can help you live a longer, healthier, and more satisfying life.

Many people my age are taking multiple pharmaceutical drugs on a daily basis, or they are impaired in some way. They have had hip replacements, knee replacements, a pacemaker, and a defibrillator. Not only that, but they also have had heart attacks and strokes, they have diabetes, and other autoimmune conditions, and they have cataracts and glaucoma. Since this is now the new norm, and they see it all around them, they have come to accept this as a normal part of aging. In response, let me tell you, it doesn't have to be that way!

I mentioned this to one of my patients and she said, "Everybody has to have something." My answer is, "Do they?"

When you ask older individuals the secret to their longevity, they will often tell you that they eat right, get plenty of exercise, and enjoy life. How are they eating differently than we are eating today? These questions can be answered by looking at the diets of many centenarians.

If you look at centenarians or supercentenarians in different parts of the world, as we will in a moment, you will notice that their diets are much different from ours. While we eat a more modern diet, they eat a more traditional diet that is free from sugars and processed foods.

> *In the end, it's not the years in your life that count. It's the life in your years.*
>
> ABRAHAM LINCOLN

ELEMENTS OF A TRADITIONAL DIET

In a traditional diet, food comes from the source. This means that the fruits and vegetables come from the ground, meat comes from the animal, and bread and other goods come from baking from scratch. Nothing comes from a factory, nothing is processed. By taking the time to ensure that we know that our food is free from chemicals and hormones, we ensure that we are putting natural elements into our bodies rather than trusting a box to tell us that the contents are healthy. Based on how "morally" other big corporations have behaved in the past, can we really trust our health to food corporations?

A hundred years ago, people ate a traditional diet because that was all there was. Everything was organic. Even though they didn't have the modern advances in medical care that we enjoy today, people lived longer and had healthier lives. Nowadays, we are seeing people die younger due to heart disease and other factors that can be directly linked to our diet. Obviously, the people who enjoyed longevity a century ago had the right idea as to what and when they ate.

According to a Weston A. Price Foundation article "Modernizing Your Diet with Traditional Foods," by Joette Calabrese, all traditional cultures:

- Consume some sort of animal protein, including organ meats and fat, every day
- Consume foods that contain very high levels of minerals and fat-soluble vitamins (vitamin A, vitamin D, and vitamin K2 found in seafood, organ meats, and animal fats)
- Consume some foods with high enzyme and probiotic content
- Consume seeds, grains, and nuts that are soaked, sprouted, fermented, or naturally leavened in order to neutralize a portion of the naturally occurring anti-nutrients in these foods
- Consume plenty of natural fats, but no industrial liquid or hardened (partially hydrogenated) oils
- Consume natural, unrefined salt
- Consume animal bones, usually in the form of gelatin-rich bone broths
- Provide extra nutrition for parents-to-be, pregnant women, breast-feeding women, and growing children, to ensure the health of the next generation
- Do not consume refined or processed foods, including white flour, refined sweeteners, pasteurized and low-fat milk products, protein powders, industrial fats and oils, and chemical additives

These are suggestions to work toward because simple, time-proven foods can make a huge difference in your health and longevity.

The trouble is, we're not eating food any more, but food-like products.

ALEJANDRO JUNGER, M.D.

ELEMENTS OF A MODERN DIET

Many people are confused, misled, or miseducated as to what constitutes a healthy diet, and assume that eliminating entire food groups like carbohydrates or protein will make them healthier, but often with dire consequences.

Let me tell you about a patient of mine who thought she was eating "healthy" because she read that eliminating animal products from your diet was much better for you.

When Greta came into my office, she complained that her once full head of hair was now falling out, and she experienced intestinal issues on occasion that were so painful that she would double over in pain.

Although she thought she was eating healthy by being a vegetarian, eschewing most animal protein and dairy, her body told another story. Upon questioning her further, I found out that she was substituting animal protein with textured vegetable proteins and various "meat alternatives" (all made from soy) deemed to be healthy (because they were sold in health-food stores), but they were nothing more than highly processed foods. Her intestinal problems came from an imbalance in intestinal flora as she ate a predominately high carbohydrate diet that did not include any fermented foods or dairy. On my suggestion, she agreed to include some animal protein and some fermented vegetables in her diet.

After she did this, her health began to improve, and her hair not only stopped falling out, but actually grew back much healthier. Now that is not to say that everyone needs to eat animal protein or everyone shouldn't be a vegetarian, because I have found that everyone needs to eat for their "condition" and constitution. These are merely guidelines.

As mentioned before, a modern diet tends to consist of more processed foods. Even if we avoid foods that we know to be processed, we are still at risk of eating foods that are harmful to our health without really realizing it. So, what are the foods that we enjoy as part of a modern diet that can be causing us harm?

Foods that we typically see in a modern diet include:

- Foods harvested from depleted soil—these foods lack the nutrients that a fertile soil can give them
- Muscle meats—while the muscle meats of animals tend to be more flavorful and filling, they lack the nutrients that the organs have to offer

- Partially hydrogenated vegetable oils
- Artificial flavors and sweeteners
- Animals that are confined and grown for food
- Pasteurized dairy products
- Canned or frozen fruits and vegetables
- Carbonated beverages and fruit juices
- Foods that are high in sugar

While some of these foods really don't seem harmful at first glance, many of them don't contain the necessary nutrients that your body needs in order to thrive. For example, an animal raised in confinement only gets the nutrients that the grower gives it. Therefore, you're getting those limited nutrients as well. If you were to eat meat from a free-range, grass-fed animal, it would be more nutritious. Not to mention all the hormones and antibiotics that are pumped into factory farm animals, which eventually end up within us.

**Really think about
what you're putting in your body.**

What if we could change how we see the foods that we eat on a daily basis? Really think about what you're putting in your body before you consume it. It may take longer for you to shop for and prepare foods that are better for you, but in the end, you will find that you will feel better and enjoy your life more. Don't eat something that you know will keep you from enjoying your life to the fullest!

We will now examine some of the world's long-lived people to find out what their secret is for increased health, vitality, and longevity, and how we can apply this to our life.

He who takes medicine and neglects his diet, wastes the skill of his doctors.

CHINESE PROVERB

THE BLUE ZONE DIET

The greatest wealth is health.

Virgil

The areas that have many people living longer and healthier lives are known as the "Blue Zones." In the Blue Zones, there are higher occurrences of people living to be a hundred years or even older. After observing the people who live in these areas, it was found that the foods that they eat and don't eat have a lot to do with their longevity.

Not only do people in the Blue Zones eat natural foods, they also make activity a normal part of their day. Taking a look at the meal of a typical centenarian from a Blue Zone, you may wonder why you haven't tried this method before. Obviously, they are doing something right in their lives in order to reach the age of one hundred. Much of our health depends upon diet and exercise. Therefore, they must eat well and exercise well. The meals that centenarians prepare and the exercise that they get are not time consuming or strenuous. They make it a natural part of their lives.

The Blue Zones include five regions in Europe, Latin America, Asia, and the United States. The people of these areas use movement to relieve high levels of stress instead of using food to ease their nerves. These people time their consumption of food so that they are not eating heavy meals later on in the day. They also move after they eat, keeping the circulation moving. Another surprising factor about their diet includes one to two alcoholic drinks daily, usually wine.

After observing these people, it was found that they have a better sense of well-being and they eat to support their body's needs rather than for comfort or convenience. People in the Blue Zones will eat foods such as lentils, beans, and other superfoods. They feed their bodies rather than feeding their appetites. The problem with many people in today's society is that they eat what tastes good rather than what their bodies really need in order to maintain optimal health.

Eating in the Blue Zone

Since the Blue Zones are found on multiple continents, there are a variety of foods that can be eaten in order to achieve this desired lifestyle.

Ikaria, Greece

Greece is known for natural and healthy Mediterranean cuisine. From garbanzo beans to wine, they have a diet that will fill them up and nourish the body. In Greece, they eat a lot of food containing lentils, honey, goat's milk, and potatoes. These foods are simple, but they contain a lot of nutrients that give the body the energy that it needs in order to work at its best. Even though Greeks eat a lot of lamb, the people on the island of Ikaria eat very little of this meat. They mainly stick to a predominately vegetarian diet.

Okinawa, Japan

In Okinawa, Japan, they eat a lot of foods that are harvested from the ocean surrounding the island. Before the mid-1900s, they ate a lot of seaweed, rice, fish, and sweet potatoes. The foods that they attribute their long life-spans to include tofu, melons, garlic, and other foods that they can harvest from the land and sea around the island.

Japan has the highest incidence of centenarians in the world.

Japan as a country has one of the highest incidences of centenarians in the world. Obviously, their diet and their lifestyles are something that we should look at closely to find what we need to do in order to live a longer and happier life.

Ogliastra Region, Sardinia

Sardinia is another region that is near the Mediterranean where people enjoy long and healthy lives. Like many people in the European countries, they drink a lot of wine and enjoy a lot of food. However, Sardinians tend to eat a lot of food that comes from the pastures. They raise goats and sheep and tend to eat a lot of goat milk and cheese. Surprisingly enough, their diets also include a lot of carbohydrates. They like to eat a lot of grains and breads.

Mediterranean diets have become extremely popular, and after looking at the people of Sardinia and Greece, we can see why. They have a balanced diet that helps them to be more active and they enjoy their lives. The foods that they eat don't make them feel tired or lethargic, but give them energy to do more.

You might think, well that's great for other countries, but what about here, in the United States. Let's take a look at the Seventh Day Adventists of California.

Loma Linda, California

There is a large population of Seventh Day Adventists who reside in the city of Loma Linda in California. They tend to live their lives from a biblical standpoint and so they don't drink, smoke, or eat processed foods. They also tend to live longer and more fulfilling lives. When questioned on their eating habits, centenarians in this region stated that they avoid activities that are common among typical Americans.

They don't watch television or other forms of common media. When they eat, they eat a diet of mainly fruits, vegetables, and grains. They won't drink anything but water and they will very rarely eat meat. By not eating anything processed, much of the population of Loma Linda are leading healthy and happy lives and living to be well past one hundred years old! But even more importantly, they remain active.

Mexico

Although we can find many people who live to one hundred or more, if they are physically or mentally impaired, they have very little quality of life. Loma Linda isn't the only place that boasts longevity in this region. In my many years of research, I have traveled to all parts of Mexico many times. In my travels, it was interesting to find that people here not only live longer, but many women never hit menopause, often having babies well into their fifties. They remained active until they were well into their nineties, and they enjoyed good health their entire lives.

I didn't see a single hearing aid, cane, or other apparatus that would indicate old age. These people were able to maintain their health and virility by eating a diet that includes beans, corn, and chili. They raised their own chickens, pigs, and goats, which provided them with their meats and cheese. Interestingly enough, they ate the whole animal, including the organs and skin. Rural people had their own herb gardens where they grew herbs that combated illness. Their snacks were fresh fruits, corn on the cob, nuts, and seeds. They obviously had found the secret to the fountain of youth!

China

In China we can observe the residents of a place called "Longevity Village," where many people not only live past one hundred but are in excellent health. What is so interesting about their diet is that they eat vegetables with every meal.

When a cardiologist Dr. John Day, from Utah, visited Longevity Village, he learned something quite fascinating about healthy living and more importantly, healthy hearts, which he now shares with his patients. When we come across long-lived people we think, oh, they have hit the genetic jackpot, but his research did not support this. In fact, his research indicated that only 24 percent of their long life was due to genes, with the other 75 percent was due to their lifestyle, including diet. He noticed that they not only ate vegetables three times per day but they also consumed fruit, nuts, seeds, legumes, and freshly caught fish. Legumes, like beans, lentils, and peas, were a main part of their diet. In Okinawa and Mexico, beans and legumes are also a daily part of the diet.

As you might recall, Dave, who had just turned one hundred in the beginning of this chapter, had a very large extended family. It turns out that he was the only one of his eight brothers and sisters who never had heart disease because he continued to eat a more traditional diet his whole life while his siblings bought into the standard American diet.

Let's look at some even more compelling research, which comes from Dr. Weston A. Price.

Old Civilizations

In the late 1920s a dentist named Weston A. Price embarked on a research mission to study those civilizations that showed supreme health from around the world. These civilizations ranged from the Inuit Eskimos, the

Masai tribes in Africa, the Australian Aborigines, to the Swiss and Gaelic people. He studied people who were still living off their traditional foods, like much of Mexico. His research is still widely respected as some of the most important research ever undertaken and here's why.

He took photographs of these people all over the world that showed the health and vitality of the individual, including their dental arches and teeth and the shapes of their faces. He was able to contrast his findings about those people eating their own traditional diet, with those who were eating a more Western, modernized, refined diet.

What he consistently found was that when a group of people strayed from their diet, overall health and the health of the mouth deteriorated, usually within a generation. He found shallower dental arches and elongated facial bone structure versus high dental arches and round or square bone structure with high cheekbones. Also, he showed that in every civilization he encountered, whenever a group of people started eating more processed grains, which lacked vitamins and minerals, their health deteriorated. The people eating the native diets rarely had any cancer, heart disease, and arthritis. They were all vibrant and healthy, from the newborn to those in their nineties. In fact, they actually looked more like the forty-five-year-olds we see in America.

Although these diets were as diversified as you would expect to find in people from Alaska to Africa, they all shared some commonalities. Most of them ate some sort of fermented foods. If they ate grains, they were whole, not processed. And all ate some sort of animal protein, legumes, fruits, and vegetables. Although much of their diet was plant based, not one of these groups were strictly vegetarian, and all included some sort of preservation, from pickling to drying.

Another commonality was that many of these civilizations did not eat muscle meats but instead ate organ meats. In these civilizations, organs were highly prized and helped them stay healthy, generation after generation. They also ate the whole animal, including bone marrow. I also noticed this during my travels in Mexico; people still eat a lot of organ meats, from intestines to brains, lungs, liver, and kidneys.

In his book *Nutrition and Physical Degeneration,* Dr. Weston Price found that these "traditional diets" contained at least four times the amounts of water-soluble vitamins and minerals than the standard American diet. In addition to that, their diet had at least ten times the amount of fat-soluble vitamins (A, D, E, and K) than ours. It is these fat-soluble vitamins that he considered to be the key catalysts behind healthy diets.

The main foods that supplied these invaluable substances were grass-fed butter and dairy, marine oils, organ meats, fish and shellfish, eggs, and animal fat. Most of these foods are considered "unhealthy" by today's standards, but they are actually very beneficial to the whole body.

What Dr. Weston Price and the Blue Zone people didn't mention is that all these cultures ate a diet that contained condiments that also brought down inflammation. Whether it was curry in India, or chili in Mexico, or ginger in China, controlling inflammation, as we mentioned in chapter one, is key to creating the proper environment that not only protects against disease, but is also crucial to healing and regeneration.

By understanding the diets of those who have found the secret to aging well, we will begin to find ways to include these healthy eating, drinking, and exercise habits into our daily routines. If you want to live a long and healthy life, the time to start making changes is now. Don't wait until your body starts to react to the choices that you are making today!

FOOD AND DISEASE

Food and what it can do for us has become a question of concern. We all think of food as a life-giving resource, but it's interesting to know that the same food that we think is giving us life can also be damaging to us.

In a modern diet, we eat many foods that are not good for us. Because of the ease of preparing processed foods, we are eating a lot of unhealthy fats and by doing this we are actually causing a lot of our own health problems. Food can be directly linked to many different diseases. Therefore, it's essential that we watch what we eat and how we eat it.

Knowing the effects of food and changing our habits are two completely different things. If we could pursue a healthier and happier existence by resetting our taste for food and taking on different habits, why don't we? Look at the centenarians that we have talked about in this chapter. They are healthy and happy individuals who enjoy what they eat. So why can't we change our habits to be more like them?

> **We've become addicted to our modern diet**
> **that is high in sugar and salt.**

The answer is a combination of factors. One reason is that we have become addicted to our modern diet that is high in sugar and salt, both of which can be very addictive. Our taste buds have gotten accustomed to high levels of sugar and salt, and so when we eat natural foods, we find them bland. But if you were to spend some time away from processed foods and take the time to get used to fresh fruits and vegetables, your taste buds will get accustomed to the subtle but satisfying taste of natural foods. Another reason is that a lot of well-meaning doctors and nutrition experts end up giving advice that is counterproductive and causes more harm than help.

Thirty years ago when I began my practice I hardly saw anyone with chronic diseases like arthritis, heart disease, cancer, diabetes, fibromyalgia, and many others. Now I see people with not just one but multiple chronic diseases, and here's why: due to our modern Western diet, people all over the world are not only fatter, but they are also sicker than ever before. Even though Japan has a very low occurrence of diabetes, obesity and diabetes are now a huge problem.

> **People in Western countries consume about**
> **150 pounds of sugar every year!**

Everywhere modern processed goods go, chronic disease including obesity, diabetes, and heart disease goes as well. Although there are a number of factors that contribute to these chronic health problems, our diet is the most important.

Over the past 160 years, our total sugar intake has skyrocketed. People in Western-diet countries are consuming about 150 pounds of sugar a year, which is over 500 calories a day of sugar!

Added sugar is a contributor to not only obesity, but also diabetes, heart disease, and cancer because sugar promotes inflammation. Worse yet is the consumption of soda and fruit juice. One study found that in children, sugar-sweetened beverages are responsible for a 60 percent increase in obesity.

People have abandoned traditional fats in favor of highly processed or hydrogenated vegetable oils. I just read a statement by a cardiologist telling people to replace butter with a canola oil spread. When health professionals blame saturated fats for heart disease, people will abandon them in favor of processed oils. However, these oils are high in omega-6 fats, which contribute to inflammation. Therefore, the misguided advice to avoid saturated fats and replace them with highly processed vegetable oils might actually be responsible for the heart disease epidemic that we see today.

Egg consumption has also decreased because of misguided advice. Eggs are one of the most nutritious foods. Although eggs are high in cholesterol, there is no evidence that they raise bad cholesterol or contribute to heart disease. As a result of this misguided advice, we have substituted refined, highly processed, and sugared boxed cereals for eggs.

Since 1950, we have decreased our egg consumption by 33 percent, while our heart disease has skyrocketed. Not only this, but people are eating more processed foods than ever before.

POINTS TO REMEMBER

Although every person has unique food preferences and needs, studies have proven that the traditional diet consistently promotes longevity and vitality.

The traditional diet is time proven. There are many people all over the world who have been eating the same way for thousands of years—look at India, Mexico, and China for proof. These people are living longer, healthier lives even today. Knowing that people are living longer due to their diets is key to understanding the message of this chapter. If you were to ask centenarians what their secret to longevity is, they would name what they eat as one of the main factors. People who eat better live longer.

I want to encourage you to think before you shop and before you eat. Now that you see that food has a direct impact upon your health, try to make the necessary changes in your diet to ensure that you don't meet a premature death due to poor eating, or a compromised old age spent hobbling between infirmaries. I encourage all who read this to try to take on a more traditional diet. Your body will thank you!

Although we can't all eat the way those people eat, here are some changes you can make right now:

- Wherever possible shop at local farmer's markets
- Buy hormone-free eggs and wild fish instead of farmed
- Buy grass-fed meats and dairy products
- Purchase foods that do not come in a package
- Try to use more natural sweeteners instead of refined sugar
- Choose whole grains instead of white flour
- Cook at home—home cooking is best; cooking with fire rather than a microwave is better
- Include seasonal and locally grown fruits and vegetables in your diet
- Include legumes, beans, nuts, and seeds
- Buy seasonal foods

Taking responsibility for our health means a commitment to change. We must be prepared to abandon lifelong habits. Most of us love our indulgences, and giving them up seems a terrible deprivation, but we cannot restore our health until we begin to place a higher value on our health than on the immediate and transient gratification that we get from certain foods.

Health is not merely the absence of disease, but it is also a state of optimum well-being from which life seems to flow effortlessly. When the body is healthy, the mind is healthy and our judgment is on target. We seem to always be "in the right place at the right time." Our intuition becomes strong and enables us to function harmoniously within our environment. The way we eat can help us enjoy life with greater health and vitality.

The first step in improving our health and vitality is to eat a diet consisting of more natural foods. Very few people can change their way of eating in a matter of days or even weeks. Each person needs a transitional period. In subsequent chapters, I will be offering recipes that will help you make this transition more easily. I hope they will inspire you to create some recipes of your own and to embrace a more natural way of eating and living. You are now on the journey to renewed health and increased vitality.

REFERENCES FOR CHAPTER 2

Gordinier, Jeff. "My Dinner with Longevity Expert Dan Buettner (No Kale Required)." *New York Times,* August 1, 2015. www.nytimes.com/2015/08/02 /fashion/dinner-with-blue-zones-solution-dan-buettner.html (accessed April 29, 2017).

Grainger, L. "Is the Blue Zone Diet the Secret to a Long Life?" *Reader's Digest Best Health,* May 2012. www.besthealthmag.ca/best-eats/healthy-eating /is-the-blue-zone-diet-the-secret-to-a-long-life/ (accessed April 29, 2017).

Johnson, Kristina. "The Live-Longer Lifestyle Plan That Really Works." *Purple Clover,* August 24, 2015. http://www.purpleclover.com/health/4232-live -longer-lifestyle-plan-really-works/ (accessed April 29, 2017).

Leyva, John. "Meet the First (and Still Best) Superfoods." HobokenFitness.com, February 13, 2014. www.hobokenpersonaltrainer.com/meet-the-first-and -still-best-super-foods/ (accessed April 29, 2017).

Michaelis, Kristen. "Traditional Diets: A Comparison." Food Renegade. www .foodrenegade.com/traditional-diets-a-comparison/ (accessed April 29, 2017).

PART 2

Your Body, Your Life

3

A GUT FEELING

No, women don't want a room of their own, women want to be able to eat whatever they want without gaining weight.

ANONYMOUS

What if we could eat whatever we want and still stay thin? What if we never got sick or depressed? What if we found a "cure" to our chronic health problems like diabetes and heart disease? What if one organ was responsible for all of this? Sounds like science fiction, but in reality this will be one of the ways we will be treated in the future. Which organ can make this happen? This organ is the intestine.

We spoke about inflammation in chapter 1, but we didn't get to speak about where inflammation begins: inflammation begins in the gut. An imbalance in the intestinal microbiome, or gut microflora, is responsible for many of our health problems. It turns out that scientists are now just discovering the power of this important organ.

It's interesting to note that most traditional cultures had some sort of fermented food or beverage in their diets. This was to maintain a healthy gut by controlling the colonies of bacteria that are essential for the functioning of the intestines. By understanding the role of the gut in illness, the future of medicine will be focused on treating illness by manipulating the intestinal flora, or bacterium. In fact, it's already happening with Crohn's disease and ulcerative colitis.

These bacteria or intestinal flora have been found to have a multifunctional use, including immunity, reducing inflammation, promoting mental and emotional health, weight control, preventing diabetes, frailty, depression, autoimmune disease, and more.

If we look at the diet of traditional cultures, we find that all of them seemed to have known about the use of fermented foods on a daily basis. They ate a diet rich in foods such as kefir, yogurt, kimchee, wine, pickles, sauerkraut, pickled vegetables, miso, and sourdough bread.

Why did they include these foods? How did they know about these foods? Interestingly, when a carnivore eats an animal, very often it is the intestines and other organs that are consumed rather than the muscle meat. Even uneducated species know the importance of eating the right parts of their prey!

Is it possible that these bacteria rule our mind? Can exercise and food choices change the intestinal microbiome? Is the gut microbiota the forgotten organ that doctors don't even address? Why does this single organ dictate whether you're healthy or sick? These are many questions that may be running through your mind right now. How can one organ dictate our entire well-being?

FAQS ABOUT THE GUT

In this chapter, we are going to answer some of these questions and figure out just why the intestines are at the center of our overall health!

What Is an Intestinal Microbiome?

You have probably heard the word *biome* come up in your education. It is a word that is used to describe a type of environment. A biome typically means that there are certain conditions present that make up an overall habitat. Just like an environmental habitat, your gut's microbiome consists of all the bacteria, fungus, and viruses that live in your intestinal tract. These all play a role in how you feel and age.

When thinking about it like this, you can probably see a lot of similarities between how your gut is feeling and the weather outside. Let me give you an example. You feel bloated and have heartburn. The spicy dinner that you just enjoyed is causing quite the stir in your digestive system. This is much like a thunderstorm in your gut. The weather moves in and changes the normal conditions of your environment.

If you can picture your gut as a habitat, you might be a little more inclined to put healthier foods and beverages into it. Thinking about the long-term effects of our present dietary decisions can really aid in making your gut feel just a little happier!

Does the Gut Microbiome Affect How We Age?

Yes. We don't realize just what a profound effect the intestinal tract has on our overall health and wellness. Not only does it affect the way we feel, but it can also predict how we age and how we feel as we grow older. The way we treat the gut now will ultimately affect the way in which it reacts later.

Aging has significant ties to our diet. Those who eat a healthier and more nutritious diet find that they look and feel better as they age. Many centenarians have reached the age of one hundred simply because they took care of their guts. They ate the right foods and pursued regular exercise. There is much to learn from our centenarian population!

Knowing that the choices we make now can ultimately affect our future should be a huge wake-up call! Try thinking about what could happen in your intestinal tract the next time you decide to eat a spicy meal or enjoy a soda. It may make you think twice about consuming the food and drink you really enjoyed before.

How Can I Tell if My Microbiome Is Unhealthy?

A study was performed where scientists observed a hunter-gatherer tribe in Tanzania. While observing their preparation of the prey, they noticed that the hunters used parts of the intestinal tract to clean the blood off their hands, and they were even seen consuming raw parts of the animal. Their connection with the natural state of the animal helped to improve their immunity. In the Westernized countries, the contact with the natural prey is so far removed that we might be setting ourselves up for disease by not having direct contact with the natural bacteria that live animals introduce. Are we impairing our health by not being closer to nature?

As I mentioned before, the intestinal microbiome holds a lot of power. It can determine how we feel, how we age, and how the body functions. We may not think about this as we eat. However, what we eat has a lot to do with the makeup of the microbiome. For some, they just know that something isn't going right in their gut. But for others, they may not even realize that there is an issue. They just associate the discomfort to what they ate. However, there is a much bigger problem going on there!

So how can you tell if your gut's microbiome is unhealthy? The common signs that there is a problem include, but aren't limited to, bloating, constipation, and incomplete and foul-smelling bowel movements that are small or shaggy and very dark in color. Also, you may experience frequent infections such as yeast and bladder infections.

We may also be jeopardizing the health of the gut's microbiome by taking antibiotics to help treat common health problems. Much of the bacteria in the gut actually aids in defending against disease, but we kill them off when we take an antibiotic!

It can be possible that you may not experience any of the common signs of an unhealthy microbiome. In such cases other factors that can help tell you whether or not you have a problem include a drastic change in behavior, onset of type 2 diabetes, obesity, and even autism in young children. These factors will not only make you feel unhealthy, but also make you look unhealthy. The skin and gut are closely related and if you have an unhealthy gut, you will also have unhealthy skin. You can see it in the form of rashes, acne, blisters, and so forth. So, if you have experienced any of the above symptoms, it may be time to find ways to change your diet.

Stress and the rise of cortisol levels can also affect the permeability of your intestinal lining, making it difficult for it to do its job properly. After a while, you will find that you are experiencing inflammation not only in your intestines, but also in other parts of your body. The toxins that cannot be filtered out of your digestive system due to poor stress management can ultimately lead to illness.

Overall, when your gut microbiome isn't healthy, you are not going to feel well. If something feels off, take a quick inventory of how your gut really feels. See if you're experiencing any of the symptoms that are listed above. If so, then it may be time for you to take some measures to cleanse your gut so that you will feel and look healthier! In the next section, we are going to look at some ways in which you can improve the health of your gut so that you can feel better.

How Can I Improve My Intestinal Microbiome?

So, you have found that your gut's microbiome really isn't doing so great. You feel bloated and it's simply not enjoyable. How can you change this in order to feel your best? In the last chapter, we discussed eating a whole-foods diet. Not only does a whole-foods diet help in your likelihood of longevity, it can also help you look and feel better on a daily basis. What you put into your body will ultimately affect the health of your gut's microbiome.

Eating for a healthier gut is a great way to clear up the unpleasant feelings. Try eating whole foods that are high in fiber and consist of plenty of probiotics. Also, try a diet that allows you to enjoy fermented foods on a daily basis. Later in this chapter, I will cover more of what a fermented food is and why it is important to the overall health of your gut's microbiome.

As in many cases, plentiful amounts of exercise can also do wonders in calming the storm of an unhealthy intestinal microbiome. Getting an adequate amount of exercise will help the flow of your intestines, keeping digestion flowing the way that it should. By mixing both diet and exercise, you will be sure to see some noticeable changes in the way that your gut feels.

THE UGLY WORLD OF CONSTIPATION

No discussion of intestinal health would be complete without mentioning constipation. We have all experienced it at one point in our lives. Practically every woman who is near or in menopause has complained of "digestive issues." This is just a polite euphemism for constipation. One woman I met related how she was constipated for a week. No matter what she tried, she still couldn't get things moving. She finally had to go to the emergency room to solve the problem. We all have our methods for treating this problem on our own. Over-the-counter laxatives are a multimillion-dollar business and yet people are still constipated. Why is this?

Much of what we consume is the primary culprit for this uncomfortable situation. How do you know that you're experiencing this not-so-lovely phenomenon? Constipation can produce irritability, sluggishness, lower back pain, bloating, and even bad breath, to name a few unpleasant side effects. Many women have told me that they were always constipated and it runs in their family. They had just come to accept it as a part of their daily lives. Why settle for this discomfort?

There is a remedy for this condition. The answer is fiber. However, you need to know which kind of fiber will treat your constipation and how to take it. Of course, fruits, vegetables, nuts, seeds, and whole grains all have fiber in them, but I have found the best fiber that produces complete bowel movements are bran, chia seeds, flax meal, and psyllium hulls. My formula is to make a shake in the morning consisting of two tablespoons of flax meal and two tablespoons of chia seeds. Blend this with your favorite beverage, protein powder, or fruit juice. At night, take two heaping tablespoons of psyllium hulls. Consuming one to three cups of coffee in the morning can also increase intestinal mobility. These methods will not only give you one excellent bowel movement, but they can also change the quality of your intestinal microbiome.

A Word about Fiber

Many people aren't aware of the role fiber plays not only in their digestive system, but also toward their heart and skin health. Fiber even improves blood sugar control and weight management. Most people need upwards of 32 grams of fiber a day, but with all the refined food people are eating, most don't get nearly close to that amount, which can be the main reason so many people suffer with constipation.

Soluble versus Insoluble Fiber

When choosing your fibers, there are two types of fibers that are important to your body. A soluble fiber dissolves in water. There are many benefits to a soluble fiber, including lowering blood cholesterol and blood glucose. An insoluble fiber won't dissolve in water. Great sources of fiber are oats, peas, beans, apples, and citrus fruits. Soluble fiber can also be found in barley and psyllium.

Why fiber? Fiber cannot be easily digested in our intestines, making it move through and produce a softer and smoother stool. Look at it as a way to aid our food through our gut and out the other side!

Some of the common foods that provide fiber that we can eat on a daily basis include:

- Oatmeal
- Fruits such as bananas, oranges, apples, mangos, and strawberries
- Beans and legumes
- Breads and grains such as dark rye and pumpernickel
- Nuts, including almonds and pistachios

Try making it a habit to include fiber in each of your meals. It will help with digestion and it will help you to avoid unpleasant constipation.

WAYS TO HEAL AND SEAL THE GUT

Now that we have talked about the gut and its unique microbiome, you might be wondering how you can make your gut the healthiest that it can be. What do you eat? What foods and beverages should you avoid? Fiber is a great way to clean out your system, but you really want to maintain a healthy microbiome all the time. Eating a whole-foods diet is just one way to help your gut heal, but there are other elements of your diet that you will want to evaluate and change.

Sugar
One thing to avoid at all costs is sugar. Sugar in your food is one way to impede the healing of your gut's microbiome. Try eating foods that use a natural alternative to sugar. As discussed in a prior chapter, sugar is one of the main culprits in inflammation, so it's best to avoid it for many reasons.

Fermented Foods
As mentioned before, fermented foods provide many beneficial elements to healing your intestinal microbiome. First of all, fermented foods provide probiotics. If you remember, having the right probiotics in your intestinal tract can help you fight illnesses that stem from the foods that

you eat. Many food-related illnesses can be avoided by having sufficient amounts of probiotics in your digestive system. Secondly, fermented foods are often consumed by those who live to be one hundred years old or more. Knowing that this is one of the basic elements of their diets, you may want to consider making it a main element in yours.

Now that we know the benefits of fermented foods, let's take a look at the types of fermented foods that you can eat right now to help start the healing process. Knowing what foods can help aid your gut's healing will give you a jump start on living a healthier and happier life. Cultures around the world still consume high amounts of fermented food on a regular basis. For example, the people of India consume a yogurt drink prior to a meal to aid in digestion. In ancient times, the Romans ate sauerkraut because of the flavor and the health benefits.

Fermented foods for healing your gut:

- Kefir, but make sure that it isn't processed and lacking live and active cultures
- Yogurt—yogurt is a great source of probiotics
- Lebne—this is a fermented product similar to yogurt but made from milk curds where the whey is discarded
- Sauerkraut
- Pickles and pickled vegetables
- Kimchi—this traditional Korean food helps to aid in immunity and provides bacteria that promotes intestinal health
- Miso, a fermented soybean paste
- Wine
- Sourdough bread
- Garlic—garlic is a great source of probiotics and helps to encourage a healthy intestinal flora
- Butter—butter provides a natural source of butyrate, which can help prevent intestine's permeability

Fiber

Along with fermented foods, fiber is a huge factor in having a balanced and healthy gut. Not all fiber is recommended for this purpose, however. We touched upon how fiber can aid in alleviating constipation, but it has other benefits besides cleaning you out. Finding which fibers will aid in healing your digestive tract will help you to feel better over time.

The importance of a high-fiber diet is indisputable. You can gain the benefits of fiber from vegetables, grains, nuts, and seeds. These foods also provide probiotics. I discussed soluble and nonsoluble fibers when we discussed constipation. They are important for the healing of your gut as well as getting rid of the toxins that are causing the indigestion and other health problems.

So, which fibers are the best for healing your gut? Fibers used for helping your digestive tract include:

- Wheat bran that doesn't contain gluten
- Psyllium hulls
- Flax meal
- Chia seeds

THE BENEFITS OF A HEALTHY GUT

Now that we have discussed how to tell if your gut is healthy and how to make it healthy, I would like to touch upon the benefits of having a healthy gut. Eating well and having great gut health can help you to see the longevity that most people hope for. By eating a balanced and healthy diet, you can heal the existing problems in your intestinal tract and allow it to aid in graceful aging. When we eat right, we are also improving our immune systems, making it less likely that we will get ill as often. No one enjoys being ill, so why not solve the problem before it even begins?

A balanced and healthy diet also reduces inflammation, which can cause many illnesses, such as heart disease, depression, diabetes, arthritis, Alzheimer's disease, frailty, and other diseases that are thought to be a result of aging. Having a healthy gut also helps the body repair and regenerate itself.

A balanced diet reduces inflammation.

With so many benefits to healing and maintaining a healthy gut, why don't we do it? It will take some lifestyle and dietary changes, but the benefits will outweigh the health problems of an unhealthy gut!

POINTS TO REMEMBER

A healthy gut can lead to many lasting benefits. Not only will it help you to look and feel better, but it will also help control inflammation and prevent disease. By making changes to your diet, exercise, and stress-management routines, you can actually help your gut to heal and remain healthy. Identifying and changing your diet and eating habits can have a huge effect on your gut's overall health.

A healthy gut can make your life much longer and more enjoyable. Making a few dietary changes can help your intestines feel better and even prevent the occurrence of disease. Your gut is the organ that controls your overall health. What you consume on a daily basis can play a huge factor in your current and future health. Why not make your dietary choices reflect how you wish to feel? Making good choices now can have positive and long-lasting effects!

REFERENCES FOR CHAPTER 3

Chutkan, Robynne. "The Questions I Get Asked the Most about the Microbiome: A Gastroenterologist Explains." *MindBodyGreen,* August 27, 2015. www.mindbodygreen.com/0-21423/the-questions-i-get-asked-most-about-the-microbiome-a-gastroenterologist-explain.html (accessed April 30, 2017).

Health Freedom Alliance. "Our Modern Lifestyle May Be Destroying Microbiome Diversity." http://www.healthfreedoms.org/our-modern-lifestyle-may-be-destroying-microbiome-diversity/ (accessed April 30, 2017).

Kellman, Raphael. "Why Fermented Foods Are Good for Weight Loss, Mood & Glowing Skin." *MindBodyGreen,* July 31, 2014. www.mindbodygreen.com/0-14758/why-fermented-foods-are-good-for-weight-loss-mood-glowing-skin.html (accessed April 30, 2017).

Marquis, David M. "How Inflammation Affects Every Aspect of Your

Health." *Mercola,* March 7, 2013. http://articles.mercola.com/sites/articles /archive/2013/03/07/inflammation-triggers-disease-symptoms.aspx (accessed April 30, 2017).

Mercola, Joseph. "Do You Really Need Poo-in-a-Pill?" *Mercola,* October 21, 2013. http://articles.mercola.com/sites/articles/archive/2013/10/21/fecal -transplant.aspx (accessed April 30, 2017).

———. "Fermented Foods: How to 'Culture' Your Way to Optimal Health." *Mercola.* http://articles.mercola.com/fermented-foods.aspx (accessed April 30, 2017).

———. "More Evidence That a High Fiber Diet Promotes Good Health." *Mercola,* October 12, 2015. http://articles.mercola.com/sites /articles/archive/2015/10/12/high-fiber-diet-promotes-good-health.aspx (accessed April 30, 2017).

Michaelis, Kristen "Reversing MS through Dietary Changes." *Food Renegade,* January 2012. www.foodrenegade.com/reversing-ms-through-dietary -changes/?utm_campaign=shareaholic (accessed April 30, 2017).

St. John, Kayleen. "10 Foods That Are Great for Gut Health." *MindBodyGreen,* August 16, 2014. www.mindbodygreen.com/0-14963/10-foods-that-are -great-for-gut-health.html (accessed April 30, 2017).

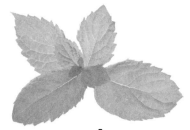

4

DETOXING THE ORGANS

The goal is to die young at a ripe old age.

Anonymous

I have come across many people in my practice and in my life who are uninterested in their health. They brush off the concept and say, "I'll eat and drink whatever I want and worry about the consequences later." One person actually said to me regarding his excessive alcohol consumption and smoking, "So I'll die two years earlier, but I'm not giving up smoking or drinking." However, what this short-sighted viewpoint fails to consider is that there are unintended consequences of such a decision that could include long-term pain and suffering, physical and mental deterioration, and other major health problems. Not to mention heartache not only for himself but also for his family and spouse.

Watching a loved one die from cancer due to years of smoking or ignoring doctor's advice, or watching the total devastation that diabetes brings can be heartbreaking. I saw my friend's husband lose the use of his hands and legs due to crippling neuropathy, and he's lucky he didn't lose a limb or become blind like so many of the farmworkers I saw when I worked in a clinic that treated the people in rural areas. I am now observing a friend losing the sight in one of her eyes due to excessive drinking. If only they had made changes to their lives earlier on, they would not be going through this pain and suffering right now.

Of course, health issues always affect more than the person afflicted. I am watching another friend go through chemo and surgeries for metastatic cancer and another drinking himself to death. Seeing so many people suffer due to things they could have changed earlier on in their lives is both frustrating and heartbreaking. Some of the people I have talked to wish they had thought about making these changes in their lives much sooner, before they became victims of crippling diseases.

> **I'd trade everything I have in a heartbeat to regain my health.**

My point is, health needs to be your priority or moved to the front burner if you value the quality of your life and also value the quality of your family's life. Health is the foundation of your life, from which everything else flows. If you don't have your health, you have nothing. I remember a very wealthy woman who was a patient of mine who came to see me in Santa Monica. She told me she was leaving for an extended vacation to Europe. I said, "That's wonderful!" However, shaking her head, she said, "I'd trade everything I have in a heartbeat to regain my health." She went on to say, "How can you enjoy your wealth or life if you are in constant pain, going to doctors all the time, and feel like a zombie from the drugs that you are put on?"

Do you want to enjoy your future? If so, then now's the time to make changes in your life that will lead to health. Putting things off until later will only prolong the issue until it's too late. I encourage you to take steps to make sure your future isn't full of health problems and heartache. In this chapter, I am going to go into detail about cleansing your most important regenerative organ, the liver. Getting rid of the toxins now can help you to feel healthier and happier later on!

HOW CAN I TELL WHETHER
I'M HEALTHY OR NOT?

You can always gauge a person's health by their eyes, skin, hair, and nails. Blood shot eyes are a sign that the liver is overworked. Pimples and other skin disorders mean the body is attempting to detox. Dull or greasy hair is indicative of your state of health. Brittle, cracking, and soft nails also tell a story. The fact is, living in today's fast-food-paced life, most of us are toxic.

> **The body's natural state is health, not disease.**

The organ of the body that bears the brunt of eliminating toxins is the liver. If you can keep your liver healthy, it can more easily perform its many functions, one of which is detoxification. You may not have realized that the liver served such an important function in your overall health. What I hope you gain from this chapter is a better understanding of how hard the liver works to cleanse your body of toxins. After knowing what it does and how to care for it, I hope you take measures to detox and keep your liver cleansed and healthy!

THE LIVER

We may not realize it, but the liver is one of the main organs that helps maintain our overall health. Since it really seems like a silent partner in our life, we really don't think about all that it does for us. Have you thought about your liver lately?

Purpose of the Liver

The liver is a super organ. There are over 500 functions that the liver performs. Some of the biggest functions it performs are to produce bile that helps in digestion, breakdown proteins, produce certain hormones, and detoxification. When it comes down to it, the liver is one giant strainer for everything that comes into your body. It cleanses your entire body. When you eat, it filters the toxins from your food. When you breathe, it filters the toxins from the air. No matter what you put into your body, the liver is responsible for filtering it.

Now, imagine if you keep throwing toxins at it. Don't you think that your liver would get tired over time? That's exactly what happens and one of the reasons people tend to suffer diseases after a life of eating and drinking things that the liver has to work hard to filter.

Even though the liver has a great regenerative quality, there is only so much abuse that it can take. That is why it is important to find ways to detox your liver regularly. By regularly, I mean daily. This can be accomplished through your dietary choices.

Why Liver Detox Is Necessary

No plan on healthy regeneration could be complete without considering the liver, which is the major detoxifying organ of the body. Every day and in every way, the body is constantly being bombarded with thousands of chemicals. These chemicals come from the food, water, and air. Sadly, these chemicals were not around fifty years ago. We have been exposed to them from the moment of birth. Somewhere along the line, this change took place in our lives and our environments.

The reason behind detoxifying the liver emanates from the concern that over a period of time, toxins are accumulating inside our bodies and brain. Some toxins are obvious, such as pesticides. Others, such as heavy metals, can be taken into the body without our knowledge. As these various toxins build over time, they can begin to not only make you feel unwell, but they also prevent the body from doing its job, which is to repair and regenerate.

> **Toxins build up inside our bodies over a period of time.**

What Harms the Liver?

Just like any other part of the body, the liver can be damaged by our environment and the things that we put inside the body. Toxins can come from a variety of sources. The food we eat and the air we breathe are just a couple of sources. If allowed, these toxins build up in our systems, and over time, we begin to feel ill. Our exterior appearance will also deteriorate, making it obvious that something isn't right.

Toxins surround us. Farmers use them to keep bugs away from our produce. Our drinking water is treated with chemicals to purify it. Ironically, it's such technological "advances" that come back to haunt us. And once a big industry is established it is very hard to change it. But the truth is that the stuff that was meant to provide us healthy food and water is actually harming us. Along with the obvious sources of toxins, there are also heavy metals that can enter our bodies and lead to liver damage. Mercury and aluminum are just a couple of examples of these dangerous substances. Also, popular pain relievers that include acetaminophen are linked to liver damage. Many popular over-the-counter medications include this compound, so be careful when taking anything that contains it!

We now know that toxins can come from food and air, but did you know that even your own body produces toxins? As the body processes occur, toxins are released into our system that require our bodies to expel them. Knowing this, you are probably thinking of ways in which you can rid your body of these little guys. One of the main ways is diet. Detoxing the liver and the digestive system can aid in improving overall health. Let's look at some foods that can help detox and aid in the health of the liver!

Foods That Help the Liver

Detoxification foods, supplements, and diets have been designed to rid the body of unwanted toxins. It's not a matter of doing a detox and then reverting back to your regular diet. One has to consume naturally detoxifying foods consistently in order to enjoy a constant feeling of health.

What can we eat or drink to aid in the health of our liver? One of the ways is by drinking warm or hot lemon water first thing in the morning on an empty stomach. Fresh lemon juice is full of things that your body needs to help with regeneration, including antioxidants, protein, vitamins, and potassium. These elements are wonderful for helping to build up your immune system and flush toxins out of your body. Drinking warm lemon water on an empty stomach helps to cleanse your system before eating or drinking anything else.

There are numerous benefits to drinking lemon water, including weight loss, better nails, decreasing the likelihood of kidney and gall stones, and boosting your immune system. Lemon juice also helps fight inflammation, a condition that signals health problems! By cleansing the body with lemon water on a daily basis, you are helping your liver detoxify your body.

Lemon juice is just a start to the ways in which diet can aid in liver detox. Below are some of the major foods that assist the body in detox.

- Cilantro for heavy metals
- Apples contain pectin, which cleans the intestines
- Avocados contain glutathione, which is essential in helping the liver to extract toxins
- Beets and beet greens are also good sources of glutathione
- Brussels sprouts are a good source of sulfur and can prevent damage by dietary and environmental toxins
- All cruciferous vegetables, such as broccoli and cauliflower, contain glucoronate, the antioxidant that promotes the production of toxin-busting enzymes
- Dandelion and other bitter vegetables like watercress aid in digestion
- Asparagus acts as a natural diuretic
- Citrus fruits contain high levels of vitamin C
- Leafy green vegetables contain chlorophyll, which absorbs many toxins—make it a practice to consume leafy green vegetables every day, even if it's in a smoothie

Eating a diet that is high in detoxifying foods can help your liver cleanse your body daily. There will be no need to do a drastic body cleanse if you learn to add these natural foods to your diet and eat them daily.

Supplements and Other Methods That Aid in Liver Detox

Along with your regular diet, there are a few other practices that can help your liver detox. As always, exercise is at the top of the list. Make it a practice to do some sort of exercise every day so that you sweat. Sweating helps release toxins through your skin, which is another way to detox the body.

While an occasional full detox will help you to feel better, what it boils down to is that eating the right foods will help your body to detox all the time, the way Mother Nature intended. Don't force your body into an unnatural emergency cleanse. Eating detoxifying foods is a much healthier way of ridding your body of unwanted toxins.

Another way to rid your body of toxins can be found in dietary supplements. Not everyone is able to get what they need from their regular diet, so supplements will aid your body in detox. The supplements I recommend include the following:

- Chlorella: a microalgae that binds to heavy metals and flushes them out of your body
- Milk thistle
- Propolis: bees use this as a sealant for their hives, but it has many health benefits in helping rid your body of heavy metals
- Alpha-lipoic acid boasts many benefits from lowering blood pressure to improving skin texture
- N-Acetylcysteine

Along with diet, supplements, and exercise, if you have access to a steam room or a sauna, use it to your benefit! This will help your body to sweat out some of the toxins it has accumulated over time!

THE INTESTINES

Along with your liver, your intestines are also responsible for ridding your body of unwanted toxins. We've already talked about the gut in the last chapter but I am mentioning it here again to talk specifically about how the intestines also help in detoxification and aid the liver in this job. Whatever you consume will make its way through your intestinal tract before being eliminated at the other end. Eating a diet that aids in intestinal detox can help aid your liver in cleansing your body of unhealthy toxins.

Intestine Detox

When we talk about detox, we often think about cleaning out the diges-tive tract. In many cases, that is true. However, the intestines are just one part of cleansing the body of unnecessary toxins. What we eat and drink are largely what will contribute to the toxins in the intestinal tract. Did you know that you could be carrying up to *twenty pounds* of toxins in your digestive system? If this statistic scares you, then you're probably eager to rid your body of these impurities. Here's how to do that.

Foods That Aid in Detoxing the Intestines

Just like eating to cleanse the liver, we can also eat to help cleanse the intes-tines. Because of the large amounts of processed foods that we eat on a reg-ular basis, our digestive tract holds on to food and toxins for much longer than is healthy. When you have too much going on in your digestive tract, you will tend to become depressed, irritable, and experience memory loss.

Eating a diet that is low in processed foods and high in fresh fruits and vegetables can help aid the process of digestion. However, if you need to clean out the toxins from your system, some foods that can help the process include:

- Fiber that is found in fruits, nuts, and other foods helps relieve con-stipation. When experiencing constipation, the digestive system will hold on to toxins longer than it should. Since it passes through the digestive system mostly intact, fiber helps keep the movement of the bowels flowing. We discussed fiber in great detail in the last chapter, so knowing that it also has cleansing benefits makes it a really good choice.
- Wheat bran
- Flax meal
- Chia seeds

HEAVY METAL DETOX

In the previous sections, I mentioned the benefits of chlorella. Chlorella is a microalgae that cleanses the system of heavy metals. Some of the main heavy metals that we encounter regularly are mercury and aluminum. These enter our bodies through what we consume and what we put on our skin. Chlorella actually binds itself to these heavy metals and aids the body in ridding itself of them. Think of it as a bouncer getting rid of unruly patrons in a club! And the best part? Chlorella can be taken in the form of a supplement! By taking it regularly, you are getting rid of heavy metals in your body!

> **Aluminum is a dangerous heavy metal that has been proven to cause cancer.**

Aluminum is a dangerous heavy metal that has been proven to cause cancer. It used to be used in deodorants until it was linked to breast cancer. The metal is a carcinogen, which deforms your cells and creates cancer cells. Cancer is not the only debilitating condition that is linked to aluminum. Aluminum can also cause dementia, Alzheimer's disease, and other cognitive problems. Since this is a common element, having ways to flush it out of our bodies is important in order to prevent the occurrence of these diseases.

Another great way to detox the body of heavy metals comes in the form of the herb cilantro. When used along with chlorella, you aren't giving heavy metals a chance to stay in your system for long. It is recommended that you use both regularly and together in order to rid your system of heavy metals. However, a word of caution concerning cilantro: consuming too much cilantro can have other digestive consequences. That is why when you use it to cleanse heavy metals, you should use it in conjunction with chlorella.

Ridding the body of toxins will produce many health benefits. Be aware, however, that the liver and the intestines are not the only organs that detox. The body is constantly detoxing itself, one organ at a time. The great thing about the human body is that it knows what is bad and what is good. It has built-in mechanisms for helping it to regenerate and stay healthy!

POINTS TO REMEMBER

Liver and intestinal detox are important because they rid the systems of harmful toxins that we consume through our diet and the environment. By taking measures to detox on a daily basis, we are giving our bodies the best chance at health and longevity. It is important to note that a detox isn't a drastic onetime deal. We can detox our bodies daily by eating foods that aid our liver and intestines in ridding our bodies of toxins.

Eating a diet containing detox foods gives the body less of a chance of holding on to toxins for unhealthy periods of time. While the health effects of toxins may not be overly obvious, they can do tons of damage to the body over time. Taking measures to cleanse will help your organs do their job more efficiently. Warm lemon water and chlorella in the detox process are natural substances that can yield great results. I encourage you to obtain and use these on a daily basis in order to give your body the chance to regenerate and repair itself.

From cancer to neurological side effects, heavy metals are a toxin that needs to be dealt with proactively. By taking measures to detox your body of heavy metals, you are insuring your future health. Toxins are not something that should be taken lightly.

While you may feel fine at the moment and see no need to change current behaviors, think about the effects that these actions can have on your future. By taking the time to detox your body on a daily basis and stopping harmful behaviors, you are giving yourself more time to enjoy life. Even if you don't care about how much time you have on Earth, remember that quality of life is an important factor. Tobacco, alcohol, and fast food not only shorten your life but also lower the quality of whatever life that remains.

Also remember that you are not the only one who will be affected by your ill health. The ones you love will also have to deal with watching you suffer. This is a heartbreaking circumstance that is best avoided.

I encourage you to make some changes to your diet to help promote cleansing and regeneration. Even though your liver isn't the first organ on your mind, think of it as still being incredibly important. Don't wear it out! Help it do its job. Take time now to promote your future health.

REFERENCES FOR CHAPTER 4

Adams, Mike. "Chlorella Detoxifies the Body by Removing Mercury and Other Heavy Metals." *Natural News,* October 30, 2009. www.naturalnews

.com/027361_chlorella_natural_detox.html (accessed April 30, 2017).

Benson, Jonathan. "Tylenol Can Kill You: New Warning Admits Popular Painkiller Causes Liver Damage, Death." *Natural News,* December 6, 2013. www.naturalnews.com/043155_Tylenol_liver_damage_warning_label.html (accessed April 30, 2017).

Devon, L. J. "Scientists Use Honey Bees' Propolis to Treat Aluminum Toxicity." *Natural News,* January 18, 2014. www.naturalnews.com/043572_propolis _aluminum_toxicity_honey_bees.html (accessed April 30, 2017).

Fassa, Paul. "Bee's Propolis Found to Combat Aluminum Toxicity and Much More." *Natural Society,* January 26, 2014. http://naturalsociety.com/bees -propolis-handles-aluminum-toxicity-much/ (accessed April 30, 2017).

Get Holistic Health. "Cilantro and Chlorella Can Remove 80 Percent of Heavy Metals from the Body within 42 Days." July 9, 2014. www.getholistichealth .com/40147/cilantro-and-chlorella-can-remove-80-of-heavy-metals-from -the-body-within-42-days/ (accessed April 30, 2017).

Health Freedom Alliance. "You Have about 20 Pounds of Poison in Your Colon. Here is What You Can Do." November 3, 2015. www.healthfreedoms .org/you-have-about-20-pounds-of-poison-in-your-colon-here-is-what-you -can-do-2/ (accessed April 30, 2017).

Kellman, Raphael. "Why Fermented Foods Are Good for Weight Loss, Mood & Glowing Skin." *MindBodyGreen,* July 31, 2014. www.mindbodygreen .com/0-14758/why-fermented-foods-are-good-for-weight-loss-mood -glowing-skin.html (accessed April 30, 2017).

Living Traditionally. "Cilantro Inflammation-Busting Recipe: Detox Your Body of Mercury and Beat Chronic Inflammation." January 07, 2015. http:// livingtraditionally.com/cilantro-inflammation-busting-recipe-detox-body -mercury-beat-chronic-inflammation/ (accessed April 30, 2017).

Louis, P. F. "Research Proven: Chlorella Protects and Detoxifies Your Liver." *Natural News,* August 2, 2013. www.naturalnews.com/041511_chlorella _liver_detoxification_superfoods.html (accessed April 30, 2017).

Mayo Clinic Staff. "Dietary Fiber: Essential for a Healthy Diet." Mayo Clinic, November 17, 2012. www.mayoclinic.com/health/fiber/NU00033 (accessed April 30, 2017).

Organic Health. "They Said That Drinking Lemon Water in the Morning Is Good for You. Here Is What They Didn't Tell You." Health Freedom Alliance, July 19, 2015. www.healthfreedoms.org/they-said-that-drinking

-lemon-water-in-the-morning-is-good-for-you-here-is-what-they-didnt-tell
-you/ (accessed April 30, 2017).

RealFarmacy.com. "16 Health Benefits of Drinking Warm Lemon Water." 2014.
www.realfarmacy.com/16-health-benefits-of-drinking-warm-lemon-water
(accessed April 30, 2017).

Toole, Michelle. "19 Super Foods to Naturally Cleanse Your Liver." *Healthy
Holistic Living,* April 21, 2015. www.healthy-holistic-living.com/19
-super-foods-naturally-cleanse-liver.html (accessed April 25, 2017).

Wright, Carolanne. "Discover the Power of Alpha Lipoic Acid for Removing
Heavy Metals, Taming Diabetes, and Protecting Against Alzheimer's."
Natural News, February 4, 2014. www.naturalnews.com/043849_ALA
_Alzheimers_heavy_metal_detox.html (accessed April 30, 2017).

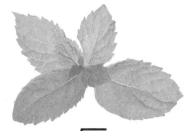

5

STRETCHING IN OUR SKINS

I'm a big believer that if you focus on good skin care, you really won't need a lot of makeup.

DEMI MOORE

Wrinkles should merely indicate where the smiles have been.

MARK TWAIN

When Barbara came for her first appointment, glancing at her consultation form, I noticed she looked a lot older than her forty-two years. She had come through a devastating divorce. She had married her high school sweetheart, worked while putting him through law school, and once he began to make some "real money," he left her for a much younger trophy wife, leaving her a single mom while the new wife enjoyed a life of incredible affluence. She was more than angry and it showed on her face. She had deep lines and furrows and wanted to know what she could do about her skin, as she was just beginning perimenopause. She also drank too much as a way of coping; she didn't exercise or get enough sleep, and ate "whatever was available at work" sometimes out of the vending machines, or a person would come by with sandwiches. Understandably, she was deeply worried about how fast her skin was aging.

If you are like most people, the first time you spotted a wrinkle, you had a tiny panic attack. Not just women, but even men care about how young they look and the first sign of aging sends everyone racing to the nearest Walgreens to buy all the anti-aging creams, lotions, or serums they can get their hands on. No matter how many over-the-counter remedies you try, nothing seems to slow the procession of wrinkles and other signs of old age. You might even have tried some home remedies such as facial exercises or herbal supplements.

You face the frustration of people advising you to eat healthy. Of course, eating healthy food and living a healthy lifestyle does help in improving your health and it does show on your skin, but it doesn't solve your problem—your existing wrinkles. The truth is that there are certain important supplements that can help you delay the signs of aging. And new techniques in skin regeneration have been developed that can help you take care of the existing signs of aging. You just have to find a good source of information that can help you understand the aging process, what factors affect your skin, what supplements and foods to eat, and which skin treatments to use. This chapter will do just that.

HOW SKIN DEGENERATES

Let's start by talking about the processes that go on behind the scenes during aging. When you understand how your body and skin ages and deteriorates, you can be better prepared to deal with it in the right way.

Aging is a natural process. There is nothing we can do to stop it. As we grow older, our bodies become weaker and that is just a fact. This is known as internal aging. Its effects on the skin include rougher skin, loose skin, skin becoming more fragile and being easily bruised, thinning of the skin, and so on. Internal aging also leads to other changes that affect the way we look. As we grow older, we lose the fat between the skin and the muscles. This leads to sunken eyes and cheeks, which gives a skeletal look. Bone and cartilage loss is also common during old age, which further changes our appearance. This type of internal aging is inevitable but we can limit the signs to a degree.

There is another form of aging that is responsible for most of our premature signs of aging. It's called external aging and the good news is that with a little bit of care, you can easily limit external aging to a minimum.

There is a difference between internal and external aging.

External aging happens when the skin deteriorates due to sun damage, air pollution, harsh weather conditions, and so on. Damage caused by lifestyle choices such as smoking, which can produce free radicals that damage cells and can lead to wrinkles, is also included under external aging. External aging can also cause precancerous lesions and eventually may even lead to skin cancer. Sun spots, freckles, and loss of collagen can all be caused due to external aging.

A lot of these factors are related to the modern lifestyle and can be eliminated by making the appropriate changes to your lifestyle. While internal aging is a fact of life, external aging is the main reason that we see premature signs of aging. Let's delve deeper into the causes of skin degeneration.

The Role of the Intestine

We've already talked about how important the intestine is but did you know that the large intestine also has a direct relationship with your skin? In fact, healthy skin is a sign of a healthy intestine. Both the skin and the intestine are boundary organs; they interact with the environment. They both help in regulating the different functions of the body by absorbing and emitting different stuff like water, chemicals, and other metabolic products. They both are organs with large surface area. And as I've already mentioned, they both help in releasing toxins from the body. When you sweat, you are releasing toxins. That's why people who use antiperspirants a lot are more prone to developing cancers such as breast cancer, liver cancer, or skin cancer, because forcing your body not to sweat traps the toxins inside.

Those who have a healthy intestine also have a soft glowing skin.

This is why if your intestine is not healthy, you are bound to have skin problems. One such example is people who suffer from a lot of acne. They often have digestive problems such as the inability to digest dairy. Processed dairy is hard to digest for humans and it ends up putrefying inside the intestine. It creates pus-filled sores inside the intestine and the same is mirrored on the skin in the form of acne.

People who have a healthy intestine often also have soft glowing skin. Try a week-long juice cleanse and you can see the results it has on your complexion. The results are not just because the juice nourishes the skin or because of the antioxidants present in the juice. The main reason is that the juice helps cleanse the digestive tract and that leads to healthier skin. Another way of achieving healthy intestine and, in turn, healthy skin is to use probiotics. Maintaining a healthy colony of gut-friendly bacteria is important for proper digestion and intestinal health.

Here's another simple thing you can do to improve both your intestine's health and your skin's complexion: drink lots of water. Water helps keep the intestine lubricated and also makes the skin cells supple and soft.

The Role of the Liver

As mentioned in the previous chapter, the liver is responsible for releasing toxins from the body. If the liver isn't healthy or is overwhelmed by a lot of toxins, the skin has to work overtime to cleanse the body. This leads to skin disorders such as dermatitis, eczema, psoriasis, itchy rashes, liver spots, hives, acne, premature aging, and wrinkling of the skin.

The conventional treatment for a lot of these skin problems includes taking strong medication and using steroidal creams and ointments. Sometimes these treatments work, but if the problem is related to an unhealthy or overloaded liver, then in the long term these drugs just introduce more toxins into the body, making the job of the liver even harder. If you have such skin problems that go away when you take medication but come back when you stop, then it might be that the root cause of the problem is bad liver health.

In order to keep your liver healthy you should supplement your diet with things that help support the liver. You can take a good liver tonic regularly, especially if you think that your liver is working overtime. Omega-3 fatty acids that are found in certain fish, fish oil, and flaxseed oil are also a good supplement for healthy liver and skin. Selenium, vitamin D, and iodine are some other supplements that you should consider to improve your liver's health. If your liver isn't healthy, your skin will show it.

The Role of Stress

We all know that stress is bad for us. But did you know that it's bad for your skin too? And I'm not just talking about the occasional zit that breaks out just before an important meeting, ironically, because of how stressed we are about the meeting. Stress can actually cause your skin to age prematurely.

Stress causes a release of adrenalin, cortisol, angiotensin, and cytokines, all compounds that can wreak havoc on your skin. Adrenalin is released when the fight-or-flight response is triggered. Originally, the fight-or-flight response was designed to help us escape dangerous situations in the wild by giving us a boost of energy and power to escape or fight predators. Our lives have changed a lot in a short span of time and we don't face life-threatening danger every day anymore. But the body's evolution doesn't happen that fast. So when we perceive a psychological threat, such as a deadline or a social gathering, our body still responds by releasing adrenalin, even though we don't really need it. Adrenalin causes the blood to drain from the extremities and be delivered to the muscles that'll help us in a fight-or-flight situation.

Cortisol, the stress hormone, can wreak havoc on your skin.

This causes an immediate washed-out look but that's not all; adrenalin then triggers the brain to release cortisol. This hormone makes the heart race and supply more blood to the muscles. If we stay stressed for a long period, then the body is always bathed in cortisol and that's not good for the skin. It breaks down collagen and can inhibit the growth of fibroblast cells, which help in generating new collagen. Without collagen, the skin becomes thin, which is a clear sign of aging.

Angiotensin releases free radicals in the body that react with the antioxidants and reduce the amount of these protective molecules in the body.

Without antioxidants, the skin gets oxidized and shows signs of aging such as spots, dullness, and wrinkles.

And finally, the cytokines cause inflammation that can damage and age the skin by damaging the collagen. It also hinders the ability of the skin to act as a barrier to external pollutants and toxins.

So stress is a big factor, especially because of the stressful life we all have today, that leads to premature aging of the skin. There are many ways of reducing stress in our lives like exercise, meditation, listening to soothing music, being grateful, spending time in nature, and the like. Now you have one more reason to use these stress busters regularly: to protect your skin.

BONUS: HOW TO TREAT SHINGLES

Shingles, or the herpes zoster virus, affects over a million people in the United States every year. This is a skin disease that leads to a severe itchy rash on the skin. It begins with a feeling of numbness and tingling along the nerve lines. The rash can turn into blisters and be very painful. Not only that, it can also lead to a problem called PHN, or Post Herpetic Neuralgia, which causes nerve pain on the affected area for years, even after the rash has been treated. This pain can vary from tenderness or numbness to unrelenting throbbing and can be very painful to live with.

The general treatment for PHN is to prescribe antivirals, antidepressants, and opiate-based pain medication. A lot of these medications only subdue the symptoms and have several side effects that can be just as bad. Shingles can also cause complications such as muscle weakness, paralysis, infections, vision and hearing problems, and so on.

Some over-the-counter medications that work for shingles are vitamin B_{12} and L-lysine, an amino acid that stops the herpes zoster virus from replicating. Shing-RELEEV is a topical cream that can also help relieve pain caused by shingles.

But the best cures for shingles are two new treatments that have worked in studies done in several labs. One is IV vitamin C. It inhibits replication of the herpes zoster virus. It has also been noted that patients suffering from PHN often have low vitamin C and so IV vitamin C helps in relieving the pain. Several case studies have shown the beneficial effects of vitamin C in improving the quality of life of patients suffering from PHN.

Microcurrent therapy is the second candidate. In this therapy, very low-level currents are used to treat the area affected by shingles. This treatment is completely safe because the electrical current used is too low to cause any damage to the skin. It helps in treating the nerve and muscle damage and reduces the pain suffered by PHN patients.

SIX FOODS FOR HEALTHY SKIN

Now that we've talked about the factors that result in skin degeneration and premature aging, let's discuss some ways you can fight these signs of aging. I've already mentioned how you can take care of your intestine and liver, reduce stress, and treat shingles, a disease that affects one in three Americans. Now, we'll talk about some other ways to keep your skin looking healthy and young. Here are six foods that you should add to your diet to maintain healthy skin.

Antioxidants and phytochemicals help fight aging directly.

Flaxseeds

Flaxseeds pack a lot of nutritional value in a tiny package. They've been used by humans as far back as the Egyptian civilization. They provide fiber, omega-3 fatty acids, alpha-lipoic acids, antioxidants, and phytochemicals. Omega-3 fatty acids are good for the liver and the skin. Alpha-lipoic acids help reduce inflammation. And antioxidants and phytochemicals help fight aging directly. There's also the fiber that keeps the intestine clean, which is also a good way to keep the skin healthy.

All of this makes flaxseeds a great supplement to include in your daily diet. Just make sure to grind the seeds before you take them because otherwise the body won't be able to digest them. Roasting them is also not such a good idea as it reduces the nutritional value of the seeds. Do remember to drink a lot of water if you are taking flaxseeds in your diet.

Avocado

Avocado is often used as a natural face mask in health spas but did you know that you can gain more benefits for your skin by eating it? Avocado is rich in antioxidants such as alpha-carotene, beta-carotene, and beta-cryptoxanthin. These antioxidants fight the oxygen-rich free radicals and protect the skin from damage. Scientific studies have also shown that these carotenoids also help in improving the skin's density, thickness, and tone.

Avocado also contains vitamins C and E. Both these vitamins help in protecting the skin from free-radical damage. Vitamin E can also help fight UV damage. Avocado also contains fatty acids such as the omega-9 fatty acids, which help moisturize the skin and keep it soft.

Coconut Oil

Coconut oil can be used as a food supplement in your diet and also as an external application on the skin. When applied directly on the skin, it helps to moisturize the skin and protects it because of its antimicrobial properties.

When used as a food supplement, coconut oil provides the body with essential fats that get stored under the skin and provide good tone to the skin. If your skin has become prematurely thin, coconut oil might be a good way to restore it to its original tone. It also contains vitamin E, which helps as an antioxidant, protects from damage, and heals damaged skin. The proteins in the coconut oil help in healing and repairing damaged tissue. You can use coconut oil as a direct supplement or use it for cooking your food.

Nuts

Nuts are a wonderful source of fiber, which keeps the intestine healthy; fatty acids, which among other things, help in reducing inflammation and swelling; and protein, which helps in repairing damage to the skin. Almonds, walnuts, and pecans are all great for the skin. It's best to eat them raw and unsalted. Make sure you eat them in moderation or they'll lead to weight gain.

Heart-Healthy Fish, Like Salmon

Salmon and other cold-water fish are rich in omega-3 fatty acids, which we've already mentioned for their awesomeness toward a glowing healthy skin. Also, salmon contains astaxanthin, which is a carotenoid and fights free radicals to prevent damage to the skin. There are a lot of other benefits of eating salmon but there is one consideration to keep in mind.

A lot of fish, especially salmon have been reported to have a high content of mercury and pesticides. Even wild-caught salmon have been found to have dangerous levels of mercury. So if you do want to include salmon and other such fish in your diet, then make sure you buy it from a reliable source. Imported salmon should be avoided as other countries might not have as strict regulations as the United States.

Chia Seeds

Chia seeds originated in Mexico and were used by the Aztecs as a quick source of energy during battle. Just like flaxseeds, they are a superfood full of nutritional value. They are rich in fiber, omega-3 fatty acids, omega-6 fatty acids, vitamin E, and protein, which help in repairing skin damage.

Apart from this, they are also a good source of minerals such as calcium, copper, potassium, magnesium, zinc, and phosphorus. Zinc helps fight acne and also keeps the skin tight and elastic. It also helps in fighting inflammation. Magnesium has a lot of health benefits such as improving blood flow, regulating blood sugar level, improving the nervous system, and more. All of these benefits help in maintaining healthy-looking skin by reducing stress and maintaining hormonal balance in the body. Potassium reduces bloating and also maintains the blood pressure. A stable blood pressure means you don't get anxious and stressed too often and, in this way, it too helps in keeping the skin healthy.

To make the most of chia seeds, soak them in water or grind them before consuming them. You can add them to drinks, salads, and other foods or just eat a spoonful between meals. They'll provide you with energy and also keep your skin healthy.

OTHER SUPPLEMENTS

Apart from these food products, there are some other supplements that you can take to encourage healthy skin and repair the early signs of aging.

Astaxanthin

Astaxanthin is the compound found in salmon and other animals such as crabs, lobsters, shrimp, and flamingoes. It turns all of these animals pink. It is derived from a type of algae that these animals feed on, called *Haematococcus pluvialis.* It is a carotenoid that acts as an antioxidant and fights the free radicals that can damage the skin cells.

> **Astaxanthin is one of the most powerful antioxidants out there.**

Astaxanthin is more powerful than other antioxidants because of certain molecular features that allow it to easily donate or accept electrons without being destroyed. Basically, the free radicals are molecules that are missing one or more electrons. They attack body cells and steal their electrons. This is known as biological oxidation. The cell membrane becomes brittle after oxidation and eventually the cell dies. When this happens to skin cells, we get signs of aging such as spots and wrinkles. Astaxanthin is very good at providing electrons to these free radicals without turning into a free radical itself.

Foods rich in astaxanthin are the best source for this supplement. You can get synthetic astaxanthin as well but its molecular structure isn't the same as the naturally occurring compound and so the benefits aren't as pronounced as that of the natural compound.

Pycnogenol

Pycnogenol is a natural plant extract that comes from the bark of a French pine tree. It contains a lot of phyto-molecules like procyanidins and bioflavonoids. All these molecules fight oxidation, membrane damage, DNA damage, inflammation, and glycation. These processes cause both internal and external aging. Pycnogenol has been found to fight all of these processes and help to slow down both external and internal aging.

Pycnogenol can fight free radicals and also protect collagen and elastin from enzymatic degradation. It can also fight UV damage and act as an internal sunscreen. UV damage of the proteins of the skin cells is one of the biggest reasons for wrinkles. Studies done on mice have found that pycnogenol reduces the amount of wrinkles on mice exposed to UV light. Several human studies have also shown that pycnogenol helps in fighting UV damage, improves skin elasticity, reduces inflammation, improves skin hydration, and reduces skin pigmentation. All this makes pycnogenol a very powerful supplement for skin care.

Hyaluronic Acid

Hyaluronic acid is a molecule that is naturally present in the skin and connective tissue in the body. It is known for its ability to hold moisture. It helps the skin stay soft and moist. It is also a good antioxidant and reduces inflammation. It also helps in healing the skin from wounds, burns, and damage from external sources. Hyaluronic acid is used as a dermal filler by plastic surgeons but it can also be used as a supplement.

A study done on the people of Yuzurihara, Japan, found that the secret of their long lives was a diet of vegetables that are rich in hyaluronic acid. The people of this area were found to have long life expectancy with 10 percent of the population over 85. Also, these people did not look as old as they were and were able to work in fields even at that ripe old age. They had both internal and external youth.

Silica

Silica is a compound that is necessary for the normal growth and maintenance of skin, hair, and nails. It helps in collagen production. Orthosilicic acid or OSA is a good supplement to help in collagen production; 5 mg of OSA, twice a day, should help in fighting the premature signs of aging. It is available as BioSil from health-food stores. A study done in Brussels, Belgium, found that women who used BioSil reported a marked improvement in skin elasticity, reduction in brittle nails, and improvement in skin repair.

MSM

MSM stands for methylsulfonylmethane. It is found in cabbage, broccoli, and brussels sprouts. It is known for its ability to soften tissue and is used as a topical cream for arthritis. It penetrates the tissue and softens the connective tissue at the joints and makes the joints more flexible. The skin also has a lot of connective tissue and MSM can help soften it up and improve flexibility of the skin.

It also helps in reducing inflammation and repairing the skin. You can use it as a topical cream. In fact it is often part of moisturizing creams as it makes the skin cells more permeable, which allows the moisturizer to hydrate more deeply. It can also be taken as an internal supplement. Drink a lot of water throughout the day when taking MSM to receive the highest hydrating benefit.

CUTTING-EDGE SKIN
REGENERATION TECHNIQUES

Michelle, a fifty-something-year-old actress had just started to feel the rejection of the youth-oriented Hollywood, as parts became few and far between. She wanted to look younger in a very competitive marketplace. She did not want a complete facelift simply because she couldn't afford the thirty to forty thousand dollars, but wanted to know what she could do to remove some of the ravages of time. I discussed with her about the latest advances in cosmetic improvements that did not involve "cutting." Living in California helped a lot since many of the top doctors who performed these noninvasive treatments also worked there.

Taking care of your diet and including supplements to improve signs of skin aging is all fine and dandy if you are still young and don't have that many wrinkles to begin with. But if you are getting old and there are plenty of signs of aging already on your skin, then just taking supplements won't help you. You'll need to go for more extreme measures.

Thankfully, the science of plastic surgery and skin regeneration has made a lot of progress in recent years. The older nip-and-tuck technique resulted in a stretched and plastic look. Now a lot of new techniques have developed that don't require highly invasive and risky surgeries. Here are some of the latest developments in skin regeneration techniques.

Stem Cell Facelift

Stem cell facelift has been created by Dr. Nathan Newman of Beverly Hills, California. In this process, a mini-liposuction procedure is first used to extract fat from the patient. The fat contains adult stem cells that usually lie dormant but when activated can turn into any type of body cell. These cells are injected into specific parts of the face where volume loss has occurred due to aging.

Since your own stem cells are being used, there are no allergic reactions. A minimum of swelling and bruising is experienced. The results can last from five to ten years and look completely natural.

Platelet-Rich Plasma

PRP, or platelet-rich plasma, is another groundbreaking skin regeneration technique. It is also known as autologous cellular rejuvenation, or ACR.

In this procedure the patient's blood is used as filler to increase the production of collagen. Because of the use of blood, it has been called the vampire facelift but what really happens is that 10 to 20 ml of blood is drawn from the patient and the platelets are extracted in a centrifuge. The platelets are then injected in specific locations in the face. They help in increasing the production of collagen and regenerate the lost volume in the face.

This technique is similar to the stem cell facelift but instead of stem cells derived from the patient's fat, platelets derived from the blood are used. Since no artificial dermal filler is used, there is no allergic or anaphylactic reaction. Minor bruising and swelling is experienced, which goes away in twelve to twenty-four hours.

Fraxel

Fraxel is a laser treatment that targets skin problems such as pigmentation, stretch marks, scars, and even wrinkles. It is different from other laser skin treatments in the fact that most laser treatments affect the entire area of the skin. This leads to a lot of bruising and a downtime of five to ten days. But Fraxel only treats small zones and so it heals much faster and the downtime is much less. Fraxel helps the collagen to regenerate and smooth out any wrinkles or scars in that area.

Hyaluronic Acid Injections

Hyaluronic acid can also be used as a dermal filler. As mentioned earlier, these molecules have the ability to hold on to water. This makes it a good injection for increasing volume. It has been on the market for a long time under popular brand names such as Juvederm, Perlane, and Restylane.

Belotero is the new hyaluronic acid that doesn't have the drawbacks of the earlier acids. It can be used under the eyes and around the mouth, areas where the older acids couldn't be used because they sometimes left a bluish hue. Voluma is another hyaluronic acid that is about to receive FDA approval and it will be the first acid that can be used to add major volume to the cheekbones and chin. Also, Restylane has been recently approved for lip revolumization.

POINTS TO REMEMBER

Skin ages through internal and external aging, which are different things. We can't do much about internal aging but we can sure as hell control external premature aging.

Skin is a very important organ when it comes to detoxification. It has a lot of similarities to the intestine and both are interconnected. A healthy intestine leads to a healthy skin. The skin can also be affected by an unhealthy liver and high levels of stress.

Whether we like it or not, our bodies will eventually get older by the natural process of internal aging. But we don't have to suffer the premature signs of aging caused by our environment and modern lifestyle. A few lifestyle changes can dramatically improve the tone and quality of your skin and also prevent further damage.

It's not just about taking care of your skin but also about adopting a wholesome approach to a healthy lifestyle because all the organs in the body are closely related to each other. The skin has a close relation to the intestine and the liver and it also reacts to stress and anxiety. By adding a few supplements to your diet you can prevent premature signs of aging. But if you want to hide the already existing signs, then modern technology has provided you with several options in the form of skin rejuvenation techniques.

REFERENCES FOR CHAPTER 5

Adams, Mike. "How Your Skin Health Reflects the Health of Your Large Intestine (and Other Holistic Principles of Wellness)." *Natural News,* June 25, 2007. www.naturalnews.com/021914_large_intestine_skin_health.html (accessed April 25, 2017).

Dawson, Alene. "Best Face Forward: If 2016 Is the Year You Improve Your Appearance, Help Is Here." *LA Times,* December 20, 2015.

Drake, Laurie Jane. "Newest Facial Fillers That Erase Lines without Surgery." *LA Times,* July 29, 2012. http://articles.latimes.com/2012/jul/29/image /la-ig-fillers-20120729 (accessed April 25, 2017).

Goins, Liesa. "What Is Fraxel?" *Everyday Health,* January 28, 2014. www .everydayhealth.com/news/what-is-fraxel/ (accessed April 25, 2017).

Graham, Rena. "Platelet Rich Plasma and Autologous Cellular Rejuvenation: A Cutting Edge Skin Regeneration Techniques." ezinepost.com. http://www .ezinepost.com/articles/article-254719.html (accessed April 25, 2017).

Janes, Beth. "Your Skin's Biggest Enemy." *HighBeam Research,* October 1, 2015. www.highbeam.com/doc/1P3-3844636681.html (accessed April 25, 2017).

Kotler, Robert. "Secrets of a Beverly Hills Cosmetic Surgeon." *WebMD,* April 14, 2011. http://blogs.webmd.com/cosmetic-surgery/ (accessed April 25, 2017).

Mercola, Joseph. "New Update: Only 4 mg of This May Help You Maintain Youthfulness." *Mercola,* May 10, 2012. http://articles.mercola.com/sites /articles/archive/2012/05/10/astaxanthin-important-key-to-slowing-agerelated -functional-declines.aspx (accessed April 25, 2017).

Miller, Zack C. "Three Keys to an Amazing Glowing Complexion." *Natural News,* January 15, 2014. www.naturalnews.com/z043519_glowing _complexion_skin_health_body_detoxification.html (accessed April 25, 2017).

Newman, Nathan. "Stem Cell Lift." Nathan Newman, M.D. http://stem-cell -lift.com/ (accessed April 25, 2017).

Norek, Danna. "Discover MSM for Soft, Deeply Hydrated and Bright Skin."

Natural News, July 2, 2013. www.naturalnews.com/041031_MSM_hydration _skin_care.html (accessed April 25, 2017).

Saint Louise, Catherine. "'Vampire Face-Lifts': Smooth at First Bite." *New York Times,* March 2, 2011.

Sarto, Janet. "Pycnogenol: Multi-Modal Defense Against Aging." *Life Extension Magazine,* August 2012.

University of Liverpool. "Face Cream Ingredient Found to Mimic Life-Extending Effects of a Calorie Restriction Diet." *Science Daily,* December 16, 2015. www.sciencedaily.com/releases/2015/12/151216231254.htm (accessed April 25, 2017).

Whitaker, Julian. "Hyaluronic Acid Benefits: Healthy Joints, Skin, and More." Dr. Whitaker. www.drwhitaker.com/hyaluronic-acid-benefits-healthy -joints-skin-and-more/ (accessed April 25, 2017).

———. "Treating Shingles Naturally." Dr. Whitaker, March 26, 2014. www .drwhitaker.com/treating-shingles-naturally/ (accessed April 25, 2017).

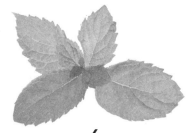

6

SLEEP
The Core of Recovery

Sleep is that golden chain that ties health and our bodies together.

THOMAS DEKKER

Sleep is the best meditation.

DALAI LAMA

When B came for her first appointment, she told me her story. She had just gotten a hysterectomy because of a fibroid tumor. When her uterus was removed she immediately went into menopause. She had not slept in a week and was starting to experience symptoms of paranoia so her doctor gave her a shot of estrogen.

She wanted to know how she could manage sleep, now that she was in menopause. She was not open to hormone replacement therapy because there was a history of breast cancer in the family. Usually bioidentical hormones applied transdermally would be a viable solution, but we needed to use a different approach.

We tried her on melatonin, because it not only helps with sleep but also lowers estrogen (which fibroid tumors feed on). I gave her a list of sleep promoting foods, including banana, turkey, oatmeal, and potatoes. I also recommended Ignatia Amara 30c at night alternating with Nux Vomica 30c, which calmed her mind. When she came back for her follow-up visit, she looked so much more relaxed. We needed to tweak her program a little bit, but basically she was much improved.

A good night's sleep is the most relaxing, blissful, and rejuvenating thing we can do to recover from the stress of daily life. But did you know that it is also one of the most essential things we do for survival? Just like food, air, and water, sleep too is a basic need for us. An average human being might sleep for one-third of his life. It might seem like such a waste of time but believe me it's not a waste at all. For if that average human was to forsake sleep and try to stay awake all the time, doing "productive" work, he would find his life shortened quite a bit.

Sleeping is not a waste of time. It is very productive. The only difference is that it's the brain and body that are being productive, while we are fast asleep, flying in and out of Neverland.

You see, when we sleep, the brain gets a break from the constant thinking, the constant absorbing, analyzing, sorting, storing, and retrieving of information. The brain puts on some soft music, lights some candles, and takes a bubble bath. But it's not like the brain stops working completely. It soon gets out of the bath and gets to work on tasks that it can't do when we are awake and it is bombarded with information. It commits information to memory. It works on problems that we can't solve while we are awake. And it looks over the repair jobs that the body is doing while we sleep.

Our bodies release hormones that help in the regeneration of cells. All the wear and tear that we suffered during the day is healed through the night. The muscles get to rest and grow. Bodybuilders know that when they are in the gym, they are not building muscles but rather breaking muscle fibers. The real growth happens when they are sleeping, as the muscles recover from the damage and become stronger to take on the extra workload. The same thing happens in the bodies of all human beings, even if they aren't involved in strenuous physical work during the day.

Sleep, quite literally, keeps us alive. Lack of sleep has been known to lead to life-threatening situations. Deprive someone of sleep for long enough, and he or she will eventually die. That's how important sleep really is. In this chapter, I'll tell you everything that you need to know about sleep, from the dangers of sleep deprivation to the tricks of sleeping better. But let's begin by talking about the benefits of sleep in more detail.

BENEFITS OF SLEEP

A recent study has proven that the brain flushes toxins during sleep. There are billions of cells in the brain. In between these cells are little channels of cerebral fluid. During the day, toxins are released from the cells and slowly build up around the cells. This is why at the end of the day we feel mentally exhausted. Our brain power is significantly reduced after a long hectic day. But when we sleep, the channels of cerebral fluid expand and allow the toxins to be flushed from the brain. So when we wake up in the morning, we feel completely refreshed and ready to tackle the tasks of the day. This might also be the reason why when we don't get proper sleep during the night, we wake up all groggy and slow.

> **Sleep can help detoxify the brain and prevent neurodegenerative diseases such as Alzheimer's disease.**

The nightly detoxification of the brain not only helps in improving brain function on a day to day basis but can also prevent diseases of the brain such as Alzheimer's disease. Certain brain toxins that have been linked with Alzheimer's are also flushed out during sleep. A study has shown that sleeping on your side leads to the maximum efficiency in flushing out these toxins by the glymphatic system.

During sleep, the brain works to store memories, which helps in improving our learning ability. Studies have shown that students who sleep well after studying a topic perform well in tests the next day because they are able to recall most of what they studied the previous day. So pulling an all-nighter to study for a big test might not be as helpful as getting a good night's sleep when it comes to doing well in a test.

A good night's sleep also helps the brain to release stress. When we are awake, we tend to obsess about the same thoughts. We worry about the future and obsess about the past. All this thinking causes stress that over time can lead to both mental and physical diseases. But by sleeping well on a regular basis we give the brain a break from these obsessive thoughts and the stress releases. That's why common wisdom says that one should "sleep on it" before making any big decision. Sleeping helps us take a step back from our thoughts. The subconscious mind works on the problem while we are asleep, and when we wake up, we can make a decision that doesn't depend on our emotional state.

Apart from these mental benefits, sleep also has some physical benefits for the body. As mentioned earlier, the body repairs the little damages suffered during the day. The muscles grow to accommodate increased workload. The lactic acid that builds up during the day in our muscles, and is the cause of muscle fatigue, is completely flushed out during the night while we sleep. The immune system gets to work and fights infections and other diseases that might be trying to attack us. The immune system also gets stronger during the night. Bad sleeping habits or lack of sleep can cause the immune system to grow weak over time and make us more vulnerable to diseases of all sorts.

The body also regulates metabolism during sleep. Sleep and metabolism are controlled by the same area of the brain. Proper sleep leads to balanced release of the hormones that control appetite and how calories are used and stored. So if we don't get proper sleep, it can also mess up our metabolism.

HARMFUL EFFECTS OF SLEEP DEPRIVATION

Another way of understanding the benefits of sleep is to look at the harmful effects that lack of sleep can have on our health. In the short term, lack of sleep can increase risk of accident. If we haven't had proper sleep for a long time, it is not advisable to do things that can cause accidents, such as driving a vehicle or operating a machine. Lack of sleep is known to cause a drop in reaction time so doing anything remotely dangerous can become even more risky.

Lack of sleep can literally kill you!

If we don't sleep properly for a long time, slowly there is a drop in neuron production in the brain. This leads to impaired brain function and cognition suffers. We can't perform even rudimentary mental tasks. Lack of sleep can also lead to mental confusion and heightened emotions.

The short-term effects of sleep deprivation are no picnic but they are nothing compared to the long-term effects. In the long term, sleep deprivation can occur due to bad sleeping habits. Sleeping fewer hours every night, insomnia or inability to sleep deeply, erratic sleeping hours, and so on, can all lead to an accumulation of effects that can be extremely harmful in the long run. In today's fast-paced world, a lot of us suffer from mild sleep deprivation without even realizing it. We survive by using stimulants such as coffee and tobacco during the day and waiting for the weekend to catch up on sleep.

This type of sleeping pattern can lead to an increased risk of heart disease and cancer. In fact, it can lead to the weakening of the immune system, which leaves us open to all kinds of diseases. Sleep deprivation can lead to inflammation in the arteries that can cause hypertension or irregular heartbeat. A study done by Emory University School of Medicine Research shows that those who frequently sleep less than six hours every night have more inflammatory proteins in their blood than those who sleep more than six hours every night. Lack of sleep can also lead to increased stress-hormone level.

Sleep deprivation can even make you gain weight. First of all, there is the simple fact that if you stay awake for more hours per day, you'll end up eating more food. Those who tend to stay awake late at night, often feel the need to snack after dinner to keep their energy level up.

Secondly, as we mentioned earlier, sleep and metabolism are controlled from the same area of the brain. Sleep deprivation can wreak havoc with the metabolism, which can lead to further weight gain. Those who suffer from sleep deprivation also tend to be more attracted to junk food. A study done by the University of Colorado at Boulder has shown that people with sleepy brains find it hard to resist cravings for calorie-rich food.

And thirdly, if you sleep less and wake up tired, you'll find it hard to exercise, which will exacerbate the other effects of sleep deprivation that cause weight gain. Lack of sleep also causes anxiety, depression, and attention deficit hyperactivity disorder (ADHD). A bad mood is another factor that can account for bad eating habits and weight gain.

Another harmful effect of sleep deprivation is premature aging. It is common wisdom that a good night's sleep helps in maintaining radiant beautiful skin. But the premature aging that lack of sleep can cause is not just limited to the superficial aspects. It can actually make you older than you are.

Simply put, aging happens when the body suffers wear and tear from within and without. And I've already mentioned that the body recovers from much of the daily wear and tear during sleep. So it is reasonable to understand that lack of sleep can lead to faster wearing of our bodies, which can cause premature aging. A study done in Great Britain found that lack of sleep was the leading cause of widespread pain in adults over fifty years of age. Widespread pain is associated with fibromyalgia.

THE ROLE OF NAPS IN REGENERATION

Up till now we've been talking about sleeping at night, but what about naps taken during the day? Studies have shown that napping during the day also has a lot of benefits. In many cultures around the world, an afternoon siesta is considered an absolute necessity but in the success-driven American culture napping is often thought of as lazy and a waste of time. Those of us who do nap in the afternoon might try to justify it by sleeping fewer hours at night so that instead of increasing our daily sleeping hours we just break it into two. But the truth is that naps of twenty to ninety minutes during the day, on top of seven to eight hours of sleep at night, can be highly beneficial.

Naps increase learning ability and memory.

Napping is a natural phenomenon and has been a part of our circadian rhythms from prehistoric times. Even if we get enough sleep during the night, it is natural for our alertness to decrease as the day goes on. For modern humans it means that our productivity decreases after lunch and we can't wait for the workday to be over so that we can go home and relax with our family and friends. But for our hunter-gatherer ancestors, mental fogginess could have led to life-threatening situations. You don't want to be yawning and feeling lazy just before a lion attacks you. So our ancestors relied on naps in the afternoon, hiding in a safe place, to refresh their brains and regain their alertness; we should do the same.

Companies like Google and Apple understand this fact and allow their employees nap time during the afternoon. It is better to take a short nap and then work with increased productivity for the rest of the afternoon than to struggle through the work with quickly diminishing alertness. We can try to use artificial stimulants like coffee or energy drinks to keep us awake but napping is the safer and healthier choice in the long run.

Naps increase learning ability and memory, give a boost to alertness, increase mental clarity, improve cognition, and aid in creativity. Not much physical regeneration can take place during a short nap but the mental regeneration and refreshment is enough to include naps in your daily routine.

You can take a nap in the afternoon, in the evening, or even at night if you are working on a nocturnal schedule. Taking several power naps during the day can also work for those who want to put in long hours of work.

Power Napping

The effectiveness of a nap depends on its duration. You should choose a duration that fits easily in your schedule and allows you to gain the kind of results you want.

Ninety Minutes

The longest nap you can take is a ninety-minute nap. Any longer and its benefits would diminish and the time spent would increase, making it unpractical. Longer naps will also cause problems with your nighttime sleeping cycle and cause more harm than benefits.

Ninety minutes is the time required for one complete sleeping cycle. This includes non-REM sleep, REM sleep (during which we dream), and deep sleep during which the body recovers. This helps in improving emotional and procedural memory and also helps in improving creativity. For someone like a musician, who uses both creativity and procedural memory while playing an instrument, a ninety-minute nap can help create highly productive evening sessions. Since the ninety-minute cycle is one complete sleep cycle, it is also easier to wake up after this nap.

Sixty Minutes

This nap is great for boosting memory; those whose work includes intense mental workouts, like scientists, can achieve a lot by taking an hour-long nap during the afternoon. But give yourself some time after waking up to clear your mind as this length of nap can lead to feeling groggy after you wake up.

Thirty Minutes

This might be the toughest nap length to pull off because just when you are about to enter the REM and slow-wave phase of the sleep cycle, you have to wake up. Hence it leads to intense grogginess after waking—for up to about half an hour. The restorative effects become clear after the first half hour but before that you might feel like you are having a hangover. So this length is best avoided if possible.

Up to Twenty Minutes

This is what is known as a power nap. It can be as short as five minutes but shouldn't be any more than twenty minutes. During the nap, you will enter only the initial stage of sleep called the non-REM sleep.

The benefit of limiting the nap to twenty minutes is that you wake up before you enter deeper sleep so it is very easy to wake up. You wake up fully reenergized and can hit the ground running and get back to work right away. You still receive the mental regenerative benefits of napping and don't have to worry about the grogginess that comes with thirty- or sixty-minute naps.

Power napping is the best way to receive the benefits of napping without having to waste too much time during the day. Most of us can find twenty minutes during the day for napping. You can even squeeze a power nap during your lunch break. While power napping, make sure that you wake up after twenty minutes and don't go into deeper sleep. Sleeping in a position where your upper body is slightly elevated, like on a recliner, can help you avoid falling into deeper sleep. The idea is to give your brain a rest without falling into deep sleep. Having a cup of coffee and then immediately taking a nap is also a good trick. The coffee takes around twenty minutes to reach your brain so by combining the effects of coffee and a power nap, you make sure that you don't fall into deep sleep.

HOW TO SLEEP BETTER

Sleeping and napping are both good for you but what if you just can't fall asleep? A lot of people suffer from sleep deficiency because they find it very hard to fall asleep. If you've spent nights lying awake in bed, watching the train of your thoughts rush through your brain, checking the clock, and feeling anxious about how few hours you have left for sleep, you know exactly what I am talking about. Sadly, a lot of us suffer from lack of sleep not because we don't value sleep but because we can't fall asleep quickly.

Luckily, there are things that you can do to ensure that you fall asleep faster and stay asleep through the night.

Supplements
There are a number of supplements that are helpful in promoting sleep.

GABA
Studies have shown that gama-aminobutyric acid (GABA), an inhibitory neurotransmitter, is responsible for insomnia. A shortage of GABA in the brain leads to low-quality sleep and insomnia. When you suffer from stress and anxiety it leads to a drop in the production of GABA in the brain. If you are anxious about not being able to sleep, it can lead to a feedback loop where your anxiety restricts GABA production and so it gets harder and harder to fall asleep. If you have been diagnosed with insomnia, you can take GABA supplements to help you sleep.

Melatonin
Melatonin is the hormone that controls sleep. It is released when the body thinks that night has arrived and we feel sleepy. Melatonin production is actually controlled by exposure to light. When the sun rises, melatonin

decreases, and when it gets dark, melatonin increases. But life has become increasingly sedentary and we stay indoors throughout the day and at night we use artificial lights. So our melatonin production is disrupted. You can take melatonin as a supplement to encourage sleep.

Although Melatonin supplement is fairly safe for use, it is not a long-term solution. You can use it to cure jet lag or to regulate sleep after night shifts but in the long term it pays to build good sleeping habits.

Magnesium

Magnesium is another supplement that can be helpful especially to those who don't respond to melatonin. Trials done on elderly patients have shown that 500 mg of magnesium taken an hour before bed can help you sleep better. This could be because a deficiency of magnesium in the body causes a reduced production of melatonin. So if you are suffering from magnesium deficiency, taking magnesium supplements can help you stabilize your melatonin production, which in turn leads to better sleep.

Magnesium L-threonate is a version of magnesium that has better bioavailability than pure magnesium. It also has known effects on improving memory so many people prefer this in place of magnesium as a supplement to help with sleeping disorders.

Jasmine Oil

While it's not a supplement, jasmine oil can also help you sleep. Studies have shown that jasmine fragrance can actually help increase GABA production and has the same effect as stronger relaxants and sedatives. All you have to do is boil a cup of water and add a few drops of jasmine oil to it and keep it at your bedside table.

Foods and Snacks

Certain foods and snacks before sleeping can also help to achieve better sleep. Oats are one such snack. Not only are they a great breakfast food but also good for eating before sleeping. They contain natural melatonin and when you have them with milk they also are a good source of tryptophan. Oats are also rich in calcium and magnesium, both of which are known to help with sleep.

Bananas are another great source of magnesium and potassium. If you suffer from muscle cramps at night and it keeps you from falling asleep, then bananas can be the perfect snack for you. The electrolytes magnesium and potassium will help relax the muscles and restrict cramps and spasms. Bananas also contain tryptophan. A research study found that bananas also help those suffering from sleep apnea by helping them keep their throats open at night and prevent any choking.

Cherries contain melatonin and having fresh cherries or drinking cherry juice has been found to help with sleep. Flaxseeds contain tryptophan and omega-3 fatty acids, which help in increasing the level of serotonin that helps regulate sleep. Omega-3 fatty acids also help in reducing anxiety and stress. Flaxseeds are also a good source of magnesium.

Other Tips

Apart from including these supplements and foods in your diet, there are plenty of other actions you can take to ensure a good night's sleep. Here are some great tips for falling asleep quickly and having a peaceful and deep sleep during the night:

- Create darkness in your bedroom by using heavy curtains and turning off the lights. If you need light for moving around at night, use red, yellow, or orange low-wattage light as it doesn't interfere with melatonin production as much as bright white and blue light.
- Expose yourself to bright daylight during the day. Fifteen minutes of sunlight exposure, especially in the morning, will help your body set its internal clock every day. This helps in producing melatonin at the right time at night. If you don't get exposure to sunlight for a long time, your internal clock can get out of sync. If someone was to be locked in a dark cave, after a while his or her body clock would not be able to regulate itself. We need sunlight to set our internal clocks.
- Don't nap for too long. Take a power nap in the afternoon but don't sleep more than that. If you have trouble sleeping at night but feel sleepy all throughout the day, it shows that your body clock has completely inverted. And to reset it, the best way is to stay awake during the day so that you feel sleepy at night.

- Go to bed at a set time and wake up at a set time every day. Stick to a routine that gives you eight hours of sleeping time. Your actual sleep will be less than that because it will take time to fall asleep and you might wake up during the night. But sticking to a strict routine helps your body adjust to the routine and it will make you sleepy at the right time and wake you up at the right time every morning, even without the need for an alarm clock.

- Exercise during the day at any time. Physical exertion helps in falling asleep. Some people feel that the exercise should not be done too close to bedtime as it prevents you from falling asleep. But any exercise, even just before bed, is better than no exercise at all. If you have a sedentary lifestyle then you must try to include some exercise during the day to ensure a good night's sleep.

- Keep the temperature of your room on the lower side. The ideal temperature for sleeping is around 60 to 68 degrees Fahrenheit. Body temperature also drops during the night, but if the room is too hot, or you are using too many blankets, the body temperature won't be able to fall and you won't be able to sleep.

- Avoid watching TV or using your computer or looking at any kind of screen for at least one hour before sleeping. The blue light produced by screens is not good for melatonin production. The body clock gets disrupted and you can't fall asleep. So create a nightly routine that helps you stay away from a screen of any kind at night before you go to sleep.

- Avoid using alarm clocks that are too loud and cause you to wake up with a jolt every morning. It is not good to wake up from deep sleep like that and it is far better to improve your overall sleeping habits so that you wake up in the morning with a softer alarm or even without an alarm at all.

- Create a bedtime routine that you follow every night before going to bed. It can be anything. Just the act of making your bed, reading in bed, or writing a journal can also work. Creating a routine means that whenever you start doing your routine, your body immediately knows that it's time for bed. You program your body to start preparing for sleep as soon as you trigger the routine.

- Turn off your phone or any other electronic device in your room. These devices create electromagnetic fields that can interfere with our brain waves and prevent us from sleeping. Those living in cities might be exposed to multiple electromagnetic fields that originate outside the house, like a transformer or power lines. You can get a gauss meter to measure the EMF levels in your bedroom to make sure that you are not being kept awake by these fields.
- Take a hot shower about an hour and a half to two hours before going to bed. The shower increases your body's core temperature, and when you get out of the shower, your body temperature drops. This drop in temperature signals the body that you are ready for sleep.
- If you can't fall asleep even after doing all of this, don't stay in bed and obsess about it. The more anxious you feel, the harder it will be to fall asleep. The best thing to do is to get out of bed and do something else, like reading a book, till you feel sleepy. Get in your bed only when you are sleepy. This helps associate the bed with sleep, and whenever you lie down on it, your brain knows that you want to sleep.

POINTS TO REMEMBER

There are a lot of benefits you get from proper and healthy sleep. And there are many harmful effects of lack of sleep, the worst one being death. Naps during the day are also important and can be a good way to make up for lack of sleep at night. A twenty-minute power nap after a cup of coffee can give you a great boost in energy and refresh your mind for the rest of the day.

If you find it hard to fall asleep, there are some simple things you can do to ensure a good night's sleep, like creating complete darkness in your bedroom, getting some sunlight in the morning, taking a hot shower, or exercising. If all of these don't work you can even choose from a variety of supplements to help you achieve the good sleep that is absolutely necessary for a healthy life.

Sleep is much more important than we think. A good night's sleep can help you deal with the daily stress of a fast-paced life. After eight hours of deep sleep you wake up rejuvenated not just mentally but physically as well. Your body is stronger and more efficient at fighting off diseases.

REFERENCES FOR CHAPTER 6

Helm, Louie. "Sleep Better with Magnesium." *Rockstar Research.* http://rockstarresearch.com/sleep-better-with-magnesium-supplements/ (accessed April 25, 2017).

Mercola, Joseph. "Could Side Sleeping Decrease Your Risk for Alzheimer's?" *Mercola,* August 20, 2015. http://articles.mercola.com/sites/articles/archive/2015/08/20/side-sleeping-may-decrease-alzheimers-risk.aspx (accessed April 25, 2017).

———. "Do You Suffer Widespread Pain? It Might Be Time to Address Your Sleep." *Mercola,* March 6, 2014. http://articles.mercola.com/sites/articles/archive/2014/03/06/poor-sleep-pain.aspx (accessed April 25, 2017).

———. "How Dangerous Is Sleep Deprivation, Really?" *Mercola,* March 27, 2014. http://articles.mercola.com/sites/articles/archive/2014/03/27/sleep-deprivation-risks.aspx (accessed April 25, 2017).

———. "The Top 5 Natural Sleep Aid Tips." *Mercola,* August 13, 2015. http://articles.mercola.com/sites/articles/archive/2015/08/13/5-natural-sleep-aid-tips.aspx (accessed April 25, 2017).

Renter, Elizabeth. "Napping Can Dramatically Increase Learning, Memory, Awareness, and More." *Natural Society,* March 17, 2014. http://naturalsociety.com/science-napping/ (accessed April 25, 2017).

Smith, Adin. "Magnesium Threonate for Sleep, Anxiety, Adrenal Fatigue and Improved Cognition." *Silicon Valley Fit,* September 8, 2012. www.siliconvalleyfit.com/blog/bid/216500/Magnesium-Threonate-for-Sleep-Anxiety-Adrenal-Fatigue-and-Improved-Cognition (accessed April 25, 2017).

Stan. "How Long to Nap for the Biggest Brain Benefits." IHeartIntelligence.com, August 29, 2014. http://iheartintelligence.com/2014/08/29/long-nap-biggest-brain-benefits/ (accessed April 25, 2017).

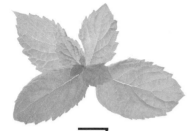

7

REMEMBERING THE BRAIN

Well, I've finally reached the wonder years . . . wonder where my car is parked? Wonder where I left my phone? Wonder where my glasses are? Wonder what day it is?

ANONYMOUS

An eighty-year-old couple was having problems remembering things, so they decided to go to their doctor to get checked out to make sure nothing was wrong with them. When they arrived at the doctor's office, they explained to the doctor about the problems they were having with their memory.

After checking the couple out, the doctor told them that they were physically okay but might want to start writing things down and make notes to help them remember things.

The couple thanked the doctor and left.

Later that night while watching TV, the man got up from his chair and his wife asked, "Where are you going?"

He replied, "To the kitchen."

She asked, "Will you get me a bowl of ice cream?"

He replied, "Sure."

She then asked him, "Don't you think you should write it down so you can remember it?"

He said, "No, I can remember that."

She then said, "Well, I would also like some strawberries on top. You had better write that down because I know you'll forget that."

He said, "I can remember that, you want a bowl of ice cream with strawberries."

She replied, "Well, I also would like whipped cream on top. I know you will forget that so you better write it down."

With irritation in his voice, he said, "I don't need to write that down! I can remember that." He then fumed into the kitchen. After about twenty minutes he returned from the kitchen and handed her a plate of bacon and eggs.

She stared at the plate for a moment and said angrily, "I *told* you to write it down! You forgot my toast!"

The human brain is the defining object that separates us from other animals. It is not the largest brain in the animal kingdom but it is pretty big for our body size. Our intelligence helped us evolve beyond the animal world and is responsible for the spectacular success of our species on this planet. It is our most precious organ and uses a large portion of the energy we generate from food.

As we grow older, just like the rest of the body, the brain is also affected. The cells in the brain, called neurons or nerve cells, slowly die off and we lose brain power. Our memory becomes weak and over time it gets harder to do even the simple things. This is the natural process of aging, and if we live long enough, we all must go through it to a certain degree.

Age-related memory loss is sometimes known by the term "senior moment," like in the joke above. Senior moments are a part of growing old and everybody has moments when they just can't remember where they put their keys or why they entered a room. But these minor lapses in memory and brain function can escalate and accumulate and lead to more serious problems that are often covered under the umbrella term, age-related cognitive dysfunction.

AGE-RELATED COGNITIVE DYSFUNCTION

As we grow older, we start becoming more forgetful, find it hard to maintain focus, and find it harder to solve problems. These are signs that brain capacity is reducing. It is a normal process of aging and for healthy individuals who have followed a healthy lifestyle throughout their life, this decline in brain capacity leads to nothing more than a few embarrassing moments. But on the other end of the spectrum, aging can lead to different types of dementia including Alzheimer's disease.

> **When your memory loss goes beyond the few embarrassing senior moments, you are in the territory of age-related cognitive dysfunction.**

This decline in brain capacity happens due to multiple factors such as:

- Free-radical oxidation damage of the brain cells
- Inflammation in the brain caused by obesity
- Insulin resistance in the brain
- Declining hormone levels
- A sedentary lifestyle that doesn't involve much use of the body and the brain
- Social isolation
- Stress
- Insufficient sleep
- Insufficient nutrition
- Imbalance of microbes in the gut, known as gut dysbiosis

We all face most of these factors to varying degrees in life and so as one gets older, one must deal with a little bit of memory loss and cognitive decline. But when these senior moments become too frequent or too severe, the person is said to be suffering from dementia.

Here are some herbs that help in fighting memory loss:

Ginkgo biloba is a tree that is found in China. It has been used in Chinese medicine for centuries. It contains flavonoids and terpenoids, which have a strong antioxidant effect. This is why it has a beneficial effect on memory and brain function. But be careful while using ginkgo supplements because they have been known to contain high levels of lead.

Bacopa is a tree that is found in India and Southeast Asia. It is known as Brahmi in Ayurvedic texts and has been used as a brain tonic for centuries. It helps in improving memory and brain function.

Reishi is known as the king of herbs and the mushroom of immortality in Eastern medicine. It has great antibacterial and antifungal properties and helps in cleaning the gut and improving the connection between the gut and the brain through the vagus nerve. It also has positive effects for immune, cardiovascular, and adrenal systems, along with the liver and nerves.

DEMENTIA

The difference between dementia and senior moments is the severity. If the person has minor lapses in memory but can still function in his or her day to day life, it's just an annoying side effect of aging but if the daily life is affected, then it can be said to be dementia. Dementia includes different diseases that all have slightly different ways of progressing but all of them lead to similar effects: these being memory loss, impaired judgment, forgetting words, loss of motor skills, and an overall decline in brain function. Dementia, depending on its type, can get worse quickly or very slowly.

Dementia is divided into different types based on the cognitive disease that causes it. Alzheimer's disease is the leading cause of dementia and amounts for about 60 percent of all cases of dementia. When a patient suffers a stroke and a lack of blood supply to the brain, it leads to the death of brain cells and is called vascular dementia. Dementia can also be caused due to Lewy bodies. Overconsumption of alcohol can lead to a type of dementia. Head injury can lead to trauma dementia. There's also a rare type of dementia known as frontotemporal dementia.

No matter what the cause, there is no cure for dementia, although certain interesting studies are being performed that hold promise in curing diseases such as Alzheimer's that lead to dementia.

When Oprah Winfrey asked her mostly female audience what they were most afraid of, she thought they would say breast cancer, but instead they answered Alzheimer's because this disease kills off brain cells and literally shrinks the brain till the patient can no longer perform even the most basic and vital functions of the body to continue living. Alzheimer's has no known cure and practically zero-percent survival rate. Normally it strikes during old age but early onset Alzheimer's can even strike as early as the forties.

The good news is that new research into the disease has found that the biggest factor in Alzheimer's might be diet related. Some researchers and doctors even call it type 3 diabetes because the damage to the brain cells is caused by the inability to process insulin. This means that if you take the time to learn about this deadly disease and make the appropriate changes to your diet while you are young, you'll considerably reduce the risk of Alzheimer's when you get old.

Let's take a deeper look into this horrible disease.

WHAT IS ALZHEIMER'S

Alois Alzheimer was a German psychiatrist who identified this disease for the first time in 1901. Before that, the patients were simply considered to have dementia. Alzheimer's disease is one of the most common forms of dementia. Over 48 million patients were reported in 2015 around the world. In America about 5.4 million people suffer from Alzheimer's. Although, there is no known cure or way of reversing the damage caused by Alzheimer's, there are some very promising protocols coming down the pipeline.

Alzheimer's is a horrible disease!

The first sign of Alzheimer's is short-term memory loss. Over time, the memory loss gets worse and the patient may find it hard to remember simple things such as common words, names of people, the date, and where she kept her things. As symptoms get worse it might lead to change in behavior and mood swings. Alzheimer's is a horrible disease because it not only affects the patient but also her family members. Alzheimer's patients become dependent on their family and require constant care. It is an emotionally and financially taxing duty and a lot of Alzheimer's caretakers report emotional problems and depression.

The mechanism behind the disease is the build up of plaque around the neurons, which hinders the connections between neurons. Amyloid beta protein is thought to be responsible for the buildup of this plaque. As the connections between the neurons decrease, the brain power also decreases. Along with this, another protein, the tau protein, is responsible for making things worse. This protein builds up inside the nerve cells and breaks the internal structure of the cell. Tiny tubes inside the nerve cells carry nutrients to the cell and tau protein breaks these tubes.

This leads to a cascading effect in the symptoms of Alzheimer's because not only are the neurons finding it hard to connect with each other, the nerve cells are also dying due to lack of nutrients. An advanced patient's brain is literally shrunken because of the death of so many brain cells. Eventually the brain can't even regulate the simple bodily functions that are vital for survival. The patient often dies due to some minor infection or disease that the body can't fight against anymore.

It is not easy to diagnose Alzheimer's early on but there are certain signs to watch out for. These signs include fatigue caused by mental tasks, depression, memory loss, and also poor digestive function.

FACTORS THAT LEAD TO ALZHEIMER'S

The cause of this deadly disease isn't fully understood. One type of Alzheimer's is dependent on genes and can lead to multiple cases in a family that has that particular gene. This is called early onset Alzheimer's because it often attacks at a much younger age than other Alzheimer's. But this gene is found in only 1 percent to 5 percent of the cases. There are a lot more theories about other factors that might be responsible for Alzheimer's. Let's discuss them one by one.

Diabetes

Diabetes is of two types. Type 1 is diagnosed in children, while type 2 is caused due to our modern lifestyle of overconsumption of sugar and fats. The body produces insulin to regulate the sugar in the body. Overconsumption of sugar leads to overproduction of insulin. This in turn leads to insulin resistance in the body and the cells don't respond well to the insulin. The body responds by producing even more insulin till finally all of the insulin in the body is exhausted and it drops to a dangerously low level.

Now researchers have found that similar processes of insulin resistance in the brain might be responsible for cognitive decline and lead to Alzheimer's. In fact, some researchers are calling Alzheimer's nothing but type 3 diabetes.

People who have diabetes have a 50 percent higher chance of getting Alzheimer's. Scientists took brain samples from nondiabetic people who had died after suffering from Alzheimer's and exposed it to insulin to measure the response of the various proteins in the cells. They found that the cells showed lower response than normal brain cells. They also found a link between insulin resistance in the brain and formation of amyloid beta plaques and tau tangles that cause Alzheimer's. In another study done at Washington University on Alzheimer's patients, they found that patients who received insulin in the form of a nasal spray were able to remember things better and had longer attention spans.

Brown University did a study on rats and found that blocking insulin from rat's brains made them forget where they were in a maze and they couldn't find their way out as easily as they could before. Another study done by Shannon Macauley from Washington University School of Medicine found that increasing the blood glucose level in rats caused an increase in amyloid beta plaque formation in the brain by as much as 20 percent in young rats and 40 percent in older rats who already suffered from Alzheimer's.

These studies have a silver lining. If Alzheimer's is related to diabetes, you can prevent it by controlling your diet. If you are still young and consciously choose a healthy diet that prevents diabetes, you can also do the same with Alzheimer's.

Sugar and Refined Carbohydrates

As we've mentioned above, even those who don't have diabetes can have insulin resistance. This is so because of our high sugar and refined carbohydrate diet. Both sugar and refined carbohydrates break down into glucose in the body and this is used to provide energy to the cells. Some scientists say that the brain functions better by burning ketones instead.

The high level of glucose in the brain leads to higher levels of insulin, which leads to insulin resistance in the brain. This can happen even if you don't have insulin resistance in the body in the form of diabetes. In order to prevent this, we need to alter our processed carbohydrate diets.

Stress

Stress is already known as a Pandora's box of diseases. Almost every disease has stress as one of the contributing factors. And if it's not a factor, stress can definitely worsen a disease. Now, studies have found that stress might lead to mild cognitive impairment, short-term memory loss, and faster aging of the brain. In this way, stress can hasten both the onset of Alzheimer's and its progression.

When you are stressed, your body releases cortisol, the stress hormone. Apart from increasing your heart rate and increasing blood flow, it also suppresses your immune system, which can lead to inflammation. Chronic stress means that your body gets used to cortisol and more of it is released, which further increases inflammation. This inflammation is linked to increased risk of diabetes, heart disease, cancer, and Alzheimer's.

By adopting a few stress-relieving techniques in your daily life, you can ensure that stress does not become the leading factor for Alzheimer's. Staying positive is important to keep stress to a minimum. Remember to smile and laugh out loud at least once daily. Exercise helps in reducing stress and also keeps the body healthy. Volunteer and help others so you can get a good perspective toward your own life and keep unnecessary stress at bay. Playing a sport or taking up a hobby is another way of busting the stress of the daily grind.

Aluminum

My mother was diagnosed with dementia at the age of eighty-three. She was put on the two standard medications for Alzheimer's: Aricept and Namenda. When there continued to be a decline in memory, mood, and function, I suggested she be tested for aluminum, and sure enough her levels were sky high.

She told me that when she was a teenager one of her teachers said she "smelled" in front of the whole class. In those days in poor families from another country, people bathed once a week, did not change their clothes every day, and no one used deodorant. Because she was publicly shamed, from that day forward she became a fanatic about using an antiperspirant (which contained aluminum).

When I saw her levels, I suggested chelation therapy, which can remove heavy metals from the body including aluminum, mercury, and lead (in those days, lead was in household paint). She refused. I then began to observe the slow but steady decline and experience the stress that Alzheimer's patients cause to everyone around them.

By the time she passed away at ninety-three, a ten-year odyssey, she not only did not recognize her family, but was also blind, couldn't talk, couldn't eat or drink, her feet became clubbed, and she was incontinent. She essentially died of starvation and dehydration. No one dies from Alzheimer's, but from what the disease causes. This is a horrible thing to witness and no one should have to experience this. She died three years ago, and that's when I began to write this book.

Aluminum is a toxic metal that is found everywhere in nature. It doesn't break down either in nature or within our bodies. Normally when we ingest aluminum, most of it is released along with other toxins. But our modern lifestyle exposes us to too much aluminum, which means that the little bits of aluminum start accumulating inside the body. When that happens, this metal can be very dangerous because the body can't get rid of it. It easily crosses the blood-brain barrier and reaches the brain where it can cause a lot of damage.

New research has shown a direct link between aluminum exposure and Alzheimer's. Those who are exposed to aluminum as an occupational hazard, for example miners and factory workers, suffer neurodegenerative diseases including Alzheimer's. Even if you are not exposed to aluminum in your workplace, our lifestyle means that all of us are ingesting much more aluminum than ever before in history.

Aluminum can enter our bodies through the following sources:

- Processed foods where aluminum is sometimes used as an additive, in foods like baking powder, self-rising flour, salt, and baby formula
- Boxed foods—even if aluminum is not used specifically, the manufacturing process of many boxed foods uses aluminum machines and the food gets contaminated with aluminum by coming in contact with the surface
- Analgesics, antacids, and some other drugs
- Vaccines—aluminum has replaced mercury in vaccines and while it's safer than mercury, it's still harmful when it gets accumulated; aluminum can actually make it harder for you to release mercury from your body by reducing production of glutathione, which helps in detoxification
- Deodorants, antiperspirants, and other cosmetics
- Aluminum products for storing and cooking food such as foil, cans, tins, and pouches

You should avoid products that contain aluminum to ensure a healthy brain and reduce the risk of Alzheimer's.

FOODS, HERBS, AND OTHER METHODS TO REDUCE THE RISK OF ALZHEIMER'S

While reducing the risk factors for Alzheimer's is a good strategy, you should also consider adding certain foods to your diet that help in reducing the risk even further.

Coffee

We all know the power of a cup of joe in the morning. Caffeine provides a boost of energy and stimulates the brain. But did you know that caffeine can also help in preventing Alzheimer's?

A study has found that coffee has a beneficial effect on type 2 diabetes. It helps in improving insulin sensitivity. This means that it can help in improving brain insulin sensitivity as well and prevent Alzheimer's. Studies have also shown that coffee works well against a lot of neurodegenerative diseases, slows down cognitive decline, and fights dementia and Alzheimer's.

This is also because of coffee's excellent antioxidant properties. The antioxidants help in fighting damage to brain cells and prevent amyloid beta plaques and tau tangles from forming.

Another study, done by researchers at Johns Hopkins University, has found that caffeine can help improve memory. Coffee also fights against Parkinson's. All this means that having one or two cups of coffee regularly can be a wonderful habit to have. Not only will it help you stay alert and productive but also fight brain damage and reduce the risk of Alzheimer's.

Coconut Oil

When the brain suffers from insulin resistance, it can't use glucose for energy. This causes the brain cells to die and leads to Alzheimer's and other neurodegenerative diseases. But there is another alternative fuel that the brain can use: ketones.

Ketones are produced when medium chain triglycerides (MCTs) are consumed in sufficient amount. These MCTs are easier to digest than long chain fats of vegetable oil and they produce ketones that the brain can use for energy even if it can't use glucose.

Coconut oil is a great source of these MCTs. Almost two-thirds of coconut oil is made up of MCTs. These benefits of coconut oil were discovered by Dr. Mary Newport who researched Alzheimer's when her husband was diagnosed with it at the age of fifty-four. He struggled with his disease and at one point it got so bad that he couldn't remember where he kept a spoon or how to get his water bottle out of the fridge. This led to a severe depression that made things worse.

Dr. Newport researched Alzheimer's thoroughly and came to the conclusion that MCTs were the best way to fight the disease because of the generation of ketones. She decided to treat him with two tablespoons of coconut oil daily for a month. In just two weeks her husband showed remarkable recovery in brain function. He recovered brilliantly and the disease did not progress further.

Her research suggests that consuming MCTs causes hyperketonemia, which leads to a 39 percent boost in blood flow to the brain. Coconut oil is the best source of MCTs as almost 60 percent of it is in the form of MCTs. It doesn't contain any cholesterol and also has omega-6 fats. Some dairy products also contain MCTs but nothing compares to coconut oil.

Cannabis

There is divided opinion in the medical community when it comes to the use of cannabis in the form of medical marijuana. There are some doctors who believe that medical marijuana might be able to fight Alzheimer's and also help patients deal with certain symptoms of Alzheimer's and side effects of standard Alzheimer's drugs. Cannabis can help fight symptoms such as depression, anxiety, insomnia, and nausea caused by medications.

Cannabis contains compounds known as cannabinoids, which have been found helpful in dealing with various symptoms of Alzheimer's. THC and CBD are two cannabinoids that have been found especially helpful. THC is the psychoactive cannabinoid while CBD is nonpsychoactive.

These cannabinoids have been found to decrease the production of amyloid beta, the protein that forms the plaques around the neurons and causes Alzheimer's. THC is the one responsible for this and it also lowers the formation of tau protein tangles. Along with this, cannabis has anti-inflammatory, antioxidant, and neuroprotective properties. Not only that, but cannabis can actually encourage neurogeneration and help in forming new brain cells.

One thing is clear, we need to conduct more studies and clinical trials to explore this protocol to fight Alzheimer's because we need any help that we can get against this deadly disease. I'll discuss cannabis in more detail in chapter 15. You'll see that it is a very beneficial herb that has been demonized unnecessarily.

Turmeric

Turmeric is a spice that has been used widely in the Indian subcontinent and Southeast Asia for thousands of years. It comes from a plant called

Curcuma longa and contains curcumin, a compound that has a lot of health benefits.

One of its health benefits is its anti-inflammatory properties. Inflammation of the brain can lead to Alzheimer's and turmeric is good at fighting inflammation. Some researchers have tried to fight Alzheimer's with pharmaceutical anti-inflammatory drugs such as ibuprofen, and although they have seen positive results at high dosage, the side effects of these drugs at such high dosage are too harmful for them to be used as a viable medicine to fight Alzheimer's. Turmeric on the other hand does the same thing without the nasty side effects. This is why in countries like India, where turmeric is a common spice in curry and is consumed daily, the cases of Alzheimer's are much rarer than in the United States.

New research has shown that not only does turmeric fight Alzheimer's by reducing inflammation but it also helps in breaking down amyloid beta plaques. This means that turmeric might even be able to *cure* Alzheimer's.

A research study done in Japan has found that Alzheimer's patients, who were given turmeric extract, regained a lot of their lost brain function and their memory improved. Further research is being carried out to confirm this finding but in the meanwhile it makes a lot of sense to include turmeric in your diet.

The problem is that American food recipes don't use turmeric as a spice. One solution can be to include Indian cuisine in your diet but a better way is to get turmeric supplements. Make sure to check that it comes from *Curcuma longa* and has curcumin.

Cilantro and Chlorella

Aluminum and other heavy metals that accumulate in the body can wreak havoc inside. Cilantro and chlorella work together as a wonderful chelating agent for heavy metals and help us flush out these toxic chemicals from the body. They bind to the heavy metals and help us release them from the body.

Cilantro is used with chlorella because cilantro is so powerful at mobilizing toxins that it can mobilize more toxins than it can carry out of the body. This can lead to retoxification of the body. But when chlorella is used along with cilantro, it acts as a secondary binding agent and helps remove all the toxins from the body. Studies have shown that cilantro and chlorella taken together can help get rid of lead, mercury, and aluminum from the body within forty-two days.

Chlorella binds to heavy metals very well. It also repairs the detoxification process of the body. It opens up the cell walls, which is necessary for the detox process. It also restores gut flora.

Cilantro too is exceptional at binding with heavy metals. It is also a good anti-inflammatory agent. It is high in magnesium, which helps in better detoxification because magnesium relaxes the arteries.

Other Foods That Help in Restoring Memory Function

While all the foods mentioned above will help you fight Alzheimer's, you might also want to consider including other foods that help in improving your memory. Here are some such foods that help in improving memory and brain function:

Garlic has antifungal properties that keep the gut healthy, but it also has anti-inflammatory properties that are great for keeping Alzheimer's at bay and improving the memory. It also reduces the risk of brain tumors.

Rosemary contains carnosic acid, which is known to fight neurodegeneration, stroke, and Alzheimer's. In fact just sniffing rosemary oil can immediately increase memory.

Olive oil is another oil that contains the good fats. It also contains hydroxytyrosol, which helps in increasing neural messaging and so improves memory and brain function.

Avocado helps in improving blood flow to the brain, which keeps the brain healthy.

Blueberries help in protecting the brain from Alzheimer's and premature aging and also improve learning skills.

Leafy green vegetables such as spinach and kale contain a lot of antioxidants that help fight free-radical damage and aging. They also contain folate, which helps in improving blood flow and decreases inflammation.

Almonds contain a protein that is known to improve production of a nerve chemical that increases memory power.

Apples contain quercetin, an antioxidant and anti-inflammatory. Most of this antioxidant is in the peel so eat the apple with the skin.

Chocolate contains flavanols, which have been found to have beneficial effects on restoring memory loss in elderly individuals. Flavanols are also found in tea and some fruits and vegetables.

Ultrasound

Researchers at the University of Queensland in Australia have recently found success in using ultrasound to treat Alzheimer's in mice. They used high-frequency ultrasound waves that do no damage to the brain tissue. It is a noninvasive procedure and moves away from the drug-based strategy to cure Alzheimer's.

The high-frequency ultrasound temporarily opens up the blood-brain barrier and activates the microglial cells that help in breaking the amyloid beta plaques and carry the toxic materials out of the open blood-brain barrier. The barrier is in place to keep bacteria out of the brain but it also locks up toxins in the brain. By temporarily opening the barrier they allow for detoxification of the brain.

By removing the amyloid beta plaques from around the neurons, a lot of the damage of Alzheimer's can be undone. The researchers have had success in 75 percent of the mice, who fully recovered abilities to find their way out of a maze, recognize new objects, and remember dangerous places they needed to avoid. The next step is to do these studies in higher animals and eventually human trials are expected to be done in 2017.

BONUS: THE MIND DIET

The MIND diet stands for Mediterranean-DASH Intervention for Neurodegenerative Delay diet. It is a hybrid diet formed by two popular diets; the Mediterranean diet and the DASH diet. These two diets have been popular for a while now as healthy diets. Studies have shown that both these diets reduce the risk of Alzheimer's.

The MIND diet combines the best features of both of these diets to specifically target neurodegenerative diseases such as Alzheimer's. Researchers have found that the MIND diet is better at reducing the risk of Alzheimer's. Even when the diet isn't followed strictly, it has a positive effect in reducing the risk of Alzheimer's.

The MIND diet includes:

- 3 or more servings of whole grains per day
- 1 glass of wine per day
- 1 vegetable per day
- 1 salad per day
- 1 serving of nuts per day
- Beans every other day
- Poultry at least twice per week
- Berries at least twice per week
- Fish at least once per week
- Use olive oil instead of other vegetable oils
- No red meat
- Less than 1 tablespoon of butter or margarine per day
- Limited amount of cheese, fast foods, pastries, and sweets as they are unhealthy for the brain

This diet was developed by nutritional epidemiologists at the Rush University Medical Center in Chicago. They conducted a study on 923 people between the ages of 58 and 98 and found that those who followed the DASH diet had a 39 percent drop in risk of Alzheimer's over a decade. Those who followed the Mediterranean diet had a 54 percent drop and the MIND diet led to a 53 percent drop in risk. The good news is that those who didn't follow the MIND diet strictly, still recorded a 35 percent drop in risk while those who didn't follow the other two diets strictly, saw no decrease in their risk of getting Alzheimer's.

This diet is not just good for the brain but for the body as well. Both the diets that are included in the MIND diet are approved by the National Institute of Health. They are great at reducing risk of heart disease and stroke, and they lower blood pressure. The longer and more consistently you can follow the MIND diet, the more benefits you'll have. And it's not a hard diet to follow, so if you can make a lifelong commitment to this diet, it will do a ton of good for your overall health and also keep Alzheimer's at bay in your old age.

SUPPLEMENTS

A diet full of brain-healthy foods will reduce the risk of Alzheimer's to a great extent. But you can take it one step further by adding supplements that have been known to fight Alzheimer's and other neurodegenerative diseases, to your diet.

Astaxanthin

Astaxanthin is probably the most powerful antioxidant known to man. We've already mentioned all about astaxanthin in chapter 5 on skincare. In short, it is the pigment that gives flamingos and lobsters and other crustaceans their pink color. But more importantly it has a molecular structure that allows it to give electrons to free radicals without becoming a free radical itself. And fighting free radicals equals fighting aging. Astaxanthin can prevent aging related neurodegeneration and dementia in this way.

It also has anti-inflammatory properties, which means it can work well for Alzheimer's. It is fat soluble and so easily passes through the blood-brain barrier. A clinical trial showed that astaxanthin improved cognition in patients. You can get a little bit of astaxanthin by eating lobsters or through krill oil but the best way to get astaxanthin is in the form of a supplement. Be sure to get a natural compound, rather than synthetic.

Galantamine

Galantamine is a natural substance extracted from flowers such as snowdrop, daffodil, and spider lily. It's an alkaloid that fights the effects of dementia, including Alzheimer's. It is also a muscle stimulant.

To understand how galantamine works you need to know about a neurotransmitter called acetylcholine. This neurotransmitter is necessary for learning and memory. Alzheimer's patients have a low level of acetylcholine. Galantamine stops the breakdown of acetylcholine and may even help in producing more of this neurotransmitter.

Galantamine has been used by the natural medicine community for a long time but now it has gotten the approval of the medical community at large, after several studies all around the world have confirmed the beneficial effects of this herbal supplement. Galantamine helps in preserving cognitive function, helps in stabilizing the behavior of the patient, and thus reduces the burden on the family and caregivers of the patient. You can get it both as a prescription drug and as a nonprescription supplement. Both contain the same thing but the supplement is much cheaper.

Lithium

High-dose lithium is used to treat bipolar disorder but there are many other benefits of lithium. One of them is that it can fight brain damage in Alzheimer's patients. Lithium is just a mineral, like sodium or potassium. While high-dose lithium requires a prescription and can cause toxic overdose, low-dose lithium is available as a supplement without a prescription and doesn't have the risk of overdose. A dose of 10 to 20 mg of lithium per day can help you keep Alzheimer's at bay.

Lithium can actually increase the gray matter as it protects and renews brain cells. Lithium limits production of amyloid beta, which creates the plaques in the brain that lead to Alzheimer's. It also prevents damage to the tau protein that forms the tangles in the brain cells that disrupt the flow of nutrients and kill the brain cells.

Lithium also helps in fighting excitotoxins such as glutamate, which have been known to cause brain damage. I've mentioned earlier the link between aluminum and Alzheimer's. Lithium helps to remove accumulated aluminum from the body.

All of this shows that lithium should be an important supplement in your diet if you want to reduce the risk of Alzheimer's. It can be taken in the form of lithium aspartate or lithium orotate, which come as 5 mg tablets and can be found in any supplement store.

Magnesium

Another mineral that works well with Alzheimer's and dementia in general is magnesium. Magnesium has been known to promote learning and memory. Research has also shown that magnesium has a beneficial effect on synaptic plasticity and density. Magnesium deficiency has been found to lead to apathy, psychosis, and memory impairment. A study done by Chinese researchers has shown that magnesium breaks down amyloid beta plaques and improves neural synapses, thus fighting Alzheimer's.

The problem has always been that normal magnesium supplements don't increase the level of magnesium in the brain. But a new compound found by MIT researchers, called magnesium L-threonate or MgT, can significantly increase the level of magnesium in the brain. MgT is much better at crossing the blood-brain barrier than normal magnesium. This is why this new supplement works well to reduce the harmful effects of Alzheimer's. You can also increase magnesium in your diet by eating more green vegetables, nuts, and whole grains.

Resveratrol

Resveratrol is an antioxidant found in grapes, red wine, dark chocolate, and raspberries. It contains polyphenols, which are good at fighting damage by free radicals. But now studies have shown that high doses of resveratrol can help prevent amyloid beta plaque buildup in the brain. Patients who took 1,000 mg of oral resveratrol showed constant levels of plaque while those who were given a placebo showed higher levels. It can also cross the blood-brain barrier with ease and has anti-inflammatory properties.

It has also been noted that the effect of resveratrol as a dietary supplement causes effects similar to calorie restriction. I've mentioned earlier that calorie restriction is a good way of slowing down the aging process. In this way, resveratrol can slow down the progress of Alzheimer's and help prevent dementia. It might also be helpful to fight against depression.

You can get resveratrol through the foods that contain it but you'd have to consume a lot of these foods to get enough resveratrol to make a difference. And we know that overconsumption of wine or chocolate isn't a good idea. Even grapes can be harmful when consumed in excess because the meaty part of the grape is almost pure fructose and can lead to diabetes. So the best source of resveratrol is as a supplement. Make sure the supplement is extracted from whole foods and not made synthetically.

Curcumin

Curcumin is the substance found in turmeric and it can be taken as a supplement as well. It has anti-inflammatory properties that have been used in Eastern medication for thousands of years. It has a polyphenolic structure similar to resveratrol, which makes it a good antioxidant as well. It can also help in breaking down the amyloid beta plaques that are the cause of Alzheimer's.

The problem with curcumin is that just because you are taking a supplement, it doesn't mean it is reaching your brain. A lot of supplements simply don't get absorbed and when they do get absorbed they don't reach the brain. When curcumin is dissolved and extracted into fat, it becomes more bioavailable to the brain. Longvida is one such supplement that attaches the curcumin to solid lipid particles. A 500 mg capsule contains about 125 mg of curcumin.

Vitamin B_{12}

Vitamin B_{12} has been found to lower the risk of Alzheimer's. You can get vitamin B_{12} from dietary sources such as liver, fish, beef, lamb, and eggs. You can also take vitamin B_{12} supplements but the results of studies done with synthetic vitamin B_{12} supplements have shown mixed results. It is better to include B_{12}-rich foods in your diet, but if you have to take supplements, you should know that oral supplements aren't as effective as injections and sublingual sprays.

Vitamin D

Vitamin D deficiency has been linked with Alzheimer's. Those who suffer from deficiency of vitamin D have twice the chance of developing Alzheimer's compared to people with normal levels. We get vitamin D from sunshine but the risk of melanoma has scared people into staying indoors. We should get at least fifteen minutes of sun exposure every day. The only other source of vitamin D is in the form of supplements. Some foods like eggs and fish contain vitamin D but only in very minute amounts.

Vitamin D helps in turning a lot of genes on and off. It helps in producing chemicals in the brain that protect the brain cells. It also helps in repairing damaged brain cells. Vitamin D has also been found to prevent type 2 diabetes. As we've seen, a very similar process happens during Alzheimer's.

When taking vitamin D as a supplement, make sure to also take vitamin K2. These two vitamins work together and help in moving calcium around the body.

Vitamin E

Vitamin E (alpha-tocopherol) has been found to slow down functional decline in Alzheimer's patients. This is just one of eight types of vitamin E and researchers say that taking a full-spectrum vitamin E supplement should be even better than taking just alpha-tocopherol.

Vitamin E can be found in nuts and green leafy vegetables and in this form you can be sure that you are getting all eight types of the vitamin. But if you have to take vitamin E as a supplement, make sure to check what type it is. Most supplements just contain alpha-tocopherol. But you should go for a full-spectrum supplement, which will contain beta, gamma, and delta tocopherol along with four types of tocotrienols.

PQQ

PQQ stands for pyrroloquinoline quinone and is a supernutrient that not a lot of people know about. This nutrient might even be part of the vitamin B family. It is found in plants, human milk, and bacteria. It is a potent antioxidant and fights damage by free radicals.

The distinguishing factor for PQQ is that it protects and can even rejuvenate mitochondria. The mitochondria are the powerhouses of the cell where the energy is generated. When free radicals damage the mitochondria, the cell dies because it doesn't get any energy. PQQ can prevent damage and also help in generation of new mitochondria. This was known to be possible only through strenuous exercise or through sustained calorie restriction. But now studies have shown that PQQ can do the same thing when taken as a supplement especially along with another supplement, coenzyme 10.

Even 20 mg per day can be helpful against damage to the mitochondria. This helps in fighting Alzheimer's too because it can protect the cells from damage due to amyloid beta and also prevent formation of amyloid beta plaques. PQQ provides overall protection to brain cells and is effective against all types of neurodegenerative diseases.

OTHER TIPS FOR PREVENTION

We've talked about foods and supplements that can help reduce the risk of Alzheimer's. But we are not done. There are a lot of lifestyle choices that can further reduce the risk of Alzheimer's and other types of dementia. If you can incorporate even a few of these in your life, it will improve your chances of never suffering through dementia. And some of these are really simple to implement.

Exercise: For a long time scientists believed that it was impossible to generate new brain cells but now it has been proven that adult neurogenesis can and does happen. One way to achieve this is by exercising. These new brain cells replace the dead cells and improve learning and memory. Studies have also shown that fitter people perform better mentally.

Avoid toxins: Processed foods such as cereals, soy, sugar, and oils often contain toxins that can damage the cells of the body. It is better for your overall health to avoid foods that contain such toxins.

Supplement diet with micronutrients: Micronutrients are vitamins and minerals and they are just as important as bigger parts of food like protein, carbohydrates, and fats. Make sure to include enough sources of micronutrients in your diet and if some nutrient is missing, take it in the form of a supplement.

Take care of your gut: We've seen how different organs of the body are related to each other. The digestive system has a strong connection with the brain. To maintain a healthy brain, you also need a healthy digestive system.

Exercise the brain: Doing mental activities such as solving puzzles or brain teasers is a good way to exercise the brain and keep it healthy. Passive sources of entertainment such as TV and movies aren't as good as active mental engagement. Even video games can help exercise the brain better than TV.

Acupuncture: Acupuncture can help increase blood flow, which helps in keeping the brain cells healthy by delivering oxygen and other nutrients to the brain and taking away the toxins.

Sleep: Our hectic lifestyle doesn't allow us to spend a lot of time on sleep. We feel that it is a waste of time. But sleep is an important need for humans. You can even call it the fourth basic need after air, water, and food. Without sleep, the brain can't recuperate from damage. Lack of sleep over long periods can hasten the deterioration of brain function.

Listen to classical music: All kind of music helps in busting stress but classical music has been found to help increase brain power.

Rosemary oil: Aromatherapy using rosemary oil can also help improve memory function.

Learn new things: Never stop learning as it helps to keep the brain healthy. Learning new skills or languages is a good way to keep dementia away.

Laugh: Laughing is a great stress buster and so can help prevent brain damage caused by the stress hormones. Some researchers have also found that laughing can actually improve memory function.

Meditate: Meditation is a great tool for dealing with stress but it has also been known to alter brain structures and improve brain function.

Avoid anticholinergic drugs: These drugs block the neurotransmitter acetylcholine, which can increase the risk of Alzheimer's. These are drugs such as nighttime pain relievers, antihistamines, antidepressants, sleeping pills, and pain relievers.

Do volunteer work: Volunteering can help you connect with others and also make you feel grateful for your life. It is a great way of busting the unnecessary stress that can arise when we get too lost in our own world. Helping those who are less fortunate than you will help you see how silly a lot of your imaginary problems are and how lucky you actually are.

Have a pet: Pets are great for relieving stress. They offer genuine companionship without the need for pretense. Pets can stimulate your brain and help fight depression and anxiety.

POINTS TO REMEMBER

An elderly widower walks into an upscale cocktail lounge. He is in his mideighties, well dressed, hair well groomed, great-looking suit, flower in his lapel, and smelling slightly of an expensive aftershave. He presents a very nice image. Seated at the bar is a classy looking lady in her midseventies. The sharp old gentleman walks over and sits alongside her. He orders a drink and takes a sip. He slowly turns to the lady and says, "So, tell me . . . do *I* come here often?"

Jokes aside, Alzheimer's is a deadly disease that is targeted to afflict 16 million Americans by 2050. And it is just one form of dementia. As we get older, we become vulnerable to different neurodegenerative diseases that can severely lower quality of life in our old age and even kill us. Alzheimer's is definitely the worst of the dementias. It doesn't have a known cure and is fatal, but what makes it even worse is that the patient has to suffer incredible loss of power and humiliation as their mental faculties slowly erode away. Not only that, the family of the patient and caregivers also suffers and they often end up with depression. It's not easy to see our loved ones slowly change into babies who can't take care of themselves.

As more studies are done on Alzheimer's, it is becoming clearer that diet and lifestyle might play an important role in the prevention of the disease and dementia in general. This is good news because it means that there are actions that you can take right now to reduce the risk of developing Alzheimer's later in life. Researchers have found that insulin resistance in the brain follows a similar process to diabetes and Alzheimer's has been even called the third type of diabetes.

Restricting sugar and processed carbohydrates in your diet and using good fats such as coconut oil can help reduce the risk of Alzheimer's significantly. Other foods, diets, and supplements can be included in your diet to fight Alzheimer's and other types of dementia, preemptively. Some exciting new protocols are showing promising results such as coconut oil, ultrasound, and cannabis.

REFERENCES FOR CHAPTER 7

Alessio, Martin. "Novel Magnesium Compound Reverses Neurodegeneration." *LifeExtension,* February, 2012. www.lifeextension.com/magazine/2012/2 /novel-magnesium-compound-reverses-neurodegeneration/page-01 (accessed April 25, 2017).

Alzheimer's Foundation of America. "What is Dementia." www.alzfdn.org /AboutDementia/definition.html (accessed May 2, 2017).

BEC Crew. "New Alzheimer's Treatment Fully Restores Memory Function." ScienceAlert.com, March 18, 2015. www.sciencealert.com/new-alzheimers -treatment-fully-restores-memory-function (accessed April 25, 2017).

Benson, Jonathon. "Turmeric Produces Mind-Blowing Recovery from Dementia Symptoms, Multiple Case Studies Show." *Natural News,* June 19, 2013. www.naturalnews.com/040858_turmeric_Alzheimers_Disease_dementia .html (accessed April 25, 2017).

Birch, Jenna. "Meet the 'MIND' Diet (It Slashes Alzheimer's Risk By 35 Percent)." *Yahoo! Beauty,* March 18, 2015. www.yahoo.com/beauty/meet -the-mind-diet-it-slashes-alzheimers-risk-113985079792.html (accessed April 25, 2017).

Block, Will. "Galantamine Combats Alzheimer's and Vascular Dementia." *Life Enhancement.* www.life-enhancement.com/magazine/article/731 -galantamine-combats-alzheimers-and-vascular-dementia (accessed April 25, 2017).

Brenoff, Ann. "Potential New Alzheimer's Treatment Fully Restores Memory: At Least in Mice." *HuffPost,* March 24, 2015. www.huffingtonpost.com/entry /alzheimers_n_6924974.html?section=india (accessed April 25, 2017).

Collins, Nick. "Alzheimer's Triggered by Type Three Diabetes." *Telegraph,* August 29, 2012. www.telegraph.co.uk/news/science/science-news/9506861 /Alzheimers-triggered-by-type-three-diabetes.html (accessed April 25, 2017).

Fassa, Paul. "Dementia Prevention: Coconut Oil Continues Succeeding; Big Pharma Keeps Failing." *Natural News,* July 20, 2014. http://www .naturalnews.com/046093_coconut_oil_low_fat_dementia_prevention .html (accessed April 25, 2017).

Gammill, Justin. "New Alzheimer's Treatment Is Fully Restoring Memory Function." IHeartIntelligence.com, October 15, 2015. http://iheartintelligence .com/2015/10/15/alzheimer-treatment/ (accessed April 25, 2017).

Georgetown University Medical Center. "Resveratrol Impacts Alzheimer's Disease Biomarker." *Science Daily,* September 11, 2015. www.sciencedaily .com/releases/2015/09/150911164211.htm (accessed April 25, 2017).

Gerard, Arielle. "An Overview of Alzheimer's Disease and Medical Marijuana." *MedicalJane,* November 17, 2014. www.medicaljane.com/2014/11/17 /alzheimers-disease-and-medical-marijuana/ (accessed April 25, 2017).

Greenfield, Beth. "Clear Link Found Between Vitamin D Deficiency and Alzheimer's Disease." *Yahoo! Beauty,* August 7, 2014. www.yahoo.com /beauty/clear-link-found-between-vitamin-d-deficiency-and-94074543072 .html (accessed April 25, 2017).

Hauser, Annie. "Is Alzheimer's a Fourth Type of Diabetes?" *Everyday Health,* September 27, 2012. www.everydayhealth.com/diabetes/0927/is-alzheimers -just-type-3-diabetes.aspx (accessed April 25, 2017).

Health Freedom Alliance. "She Gave Her Husband 1 Tbsp of Coconut Oil Twice a Day for a Month. You Won't Believe What Happened!" January 1, 2016. www.healthfreedoms.org/she-gave-her-husband-1-tbsp-of-coconut-oil -twice-a-day-for-a-month-you-wont-believe-what-happened/ (accessed April 25, 2017).

The Hearty Soul. "Immediately Improve Brain Function by Taking 2.7 Tablespoons of Coconut Oil. Here's How." August 21, 2015. http:// theheartysoul.com/coconut-oil-for-brain-function/ (accessed April 25, 2017).

Helms, Jana. "Interview with Dr. Christopher Ochner of the Alzheimer's Diet." Alzheimers.net, October 21, 2013. www.alzheimers.net/2013-10-21/dr -ochner-alzheimers-diet/ (accessed April 25, 2017).

Henry, Derek. "Four Herbs That Boost Your Brain Capacity." *Natural News,* June 5, 2014. www.naturalnews.com/045442_herbal_medicine_brain _function_Ginkgo_biloba.html (accessed April 25, 2017).

IOS Press, "Can Physical Exercise Enhance Long Term Memory?" *Science Daily,* November 25, 2015. www.sciencedaily.com/releases/2015/11/151125104750 .htm (accessed April 25, 2017).

Jockers, David. "Boost Your Brain-Regenerative Capabilities with Unique Supplemental Compounds." *Natural News,* October 25, 2014. www .naturalnews.com/047390_brain_regeneration_supplements_essential _nutrients.html (accessed April 25, 2017).

Johns Hopkins University. "It's All Coming Back to Me Now: Researchers Find Caffeine Enhances Memory." *Science Daily,* January 12, 2014. www

.sciencedaily.com/releases/2014/01/140112190725.htm (accessed April 25, 2017).

Kardon, Sherice. "Brain Diet: 10 Foods That Sharpen Memory and Boost Memory Function." *Natural News Blogs,* October 13, 2015. http://blogs .naturalnews.com/brain-diet-10-foods-sharpen-memory-boost-memory -function/ (accessed April 25, 2017).

Kresser, Chris. "How to Prevent Spending the Last 10 Years of Your Life in a Diaper and a Wheelchair." ChrisKresser.com, January 10, 2014. https:// chriskresser.com/how-to-prevent-spending-the-last-10-years-of-your-life-in -a-diaper-and-a-wheelchair/ (accessed April 25, 2017).

Longevity-and-Antiaging-Secrets.com. "Mitochondrial Biogenesis: Rejuvenate Your Cells with PQQ." www.longevity-and-antiaging-secrets.com /mitochondrial-biogenesis.html (accessed April 25, 2017).

Lucille, Holly. "Turmeric and Alzheimer's Disease." *American College for Advancement in Medicine,* August 23, 2010. www.acam.org/blogpost/1092863 /185793/Tumeric-and-Alzheimer-s-Disease (accessed April 25, 2017).

Menard, Kim. "Brain Insulin Resistance Contributes to Cognitive Decline in Alzheimer's Disease." *Penn Medicine News,* March 23, 2012. www.uphs.upenn .edu/news/News_Releases/2012/03/insulin/ (accessed April 25, 2017).

Mercola, Joseph. "Alzheimer's: A Disease Fed by Sugar." *Mercola,* August 13, 2015. http://articles.mercola.com/sites/articles/archive/2015/08/13/sugar -alzheimers-disease-link.aspx (accessed April 25, 2017).

———. "Alzheimer's Disease: Yes, It's Preventable!" *Mercola,* May 22, 2014. http://articles.mercola.com/sites/articles/archive/2014/05/22/alzheimers -disease-prevention.aspx (accessed April 25, 2017).

———. "Astaxanthin: A Rising Star in Alzheimer's Prevention." *Mercola,* July 1, 2012. http://articles.mercola.com/sites/articles/archive/2012/07/01 /astaxanthin-for-dementia.aspx (accessed April 25, 2017).

———. "Easy Ways to Boost Your Ability to Recall Now: And Later." *Mercola,* October 22, 2015. http://articles.mercola.com/sites/articles /archive/2015/10/22/ways-to-boost-memory.aspx (accessed April 25, 2017).

———. "First Case Study to Show Direct Link Between Alzheimer's and Aluminum Toxicity." *Mercola,* March 22, 2014. http://articles.mercola .com/sites/articles/archive/2014/03/22/aluminum-toxicity-alzheimers.aspx (accessed April 25, 2017).

———. "How Sugar Harms Your Brain Health and Drives Alzheimer's

Epidemic." *Mercola,* July 24, 2014. http://articles.mercola.com/sites/articles /archive/2014/07/24/sugar-brain-function.aspx (accessed April 25, 2017).

———. "Resveratrol May Offer Protection Against Alzheimer's." *Mercola,* September 28, 2015. http://articles.mercola.com/sites/articles/archive/2015 /09/28/resveratrol-alzheimers-disease.aspx (accessed April 25, 2017).

———. "Stress Promotes Memory Decline and Dementia Later in Life." *Mercola,* July 3, 2014. http://articles.mercola.com/sites/articles/archive/2014/07/03 /stress-memory-loss.aspx (accessed April 25, 2017).

———. "Vitamin B$_{12}$: The Best Kept Secret for Avoiding Alzheimer's." *Mercola,* November 19, 2010. http://articles.mercola.com/sites/articles /archive/2010/11/19/vitamin-b12-helps-ward-off-alzheimers.aspx (accessed April 25, 2017).

———. "Vitamin D for Depression, Dementia and Diabetes." *Mercola,* August 21, 2014. http://articles.mercola.com/sites/articles/archive/2014/08/21/vitamin -d-depression-dementia.aspx (accessed April 25, 2017).

———. "Vitamin E May Offer Benefits to Alzheimer's Patients." *Mercola,* January 23, 2014. http://articles.mercola.com/sites/articles/archive/2014/01/23/vitamin -e-alzheimers-disease.aspx (accessed April 25, 2017).

Napoletan, Ann. "Can Coconut Oil Prevent Alzheimer's?" Alzheimers.net, August 20, 2014. www.alzheimers.net/2013-05-29/coconut-oil-for-alzheimers (accessed April 25, 2017).

Phillip, John. "B Vitamins Help Reduce Brain Shrinkage and May Prevent Alzheimer's Disease." *Natural News,* June 8, 2013. www.naturalnews .com/040689_dementia_Alzheimers_disease_vitamin_B.html (accessed April 25, 2017).

Richards, Karen Lee. "Rejuvenating the Brain: How PQQ Helps Power Up Mental Processing." *ProHealth,* March 30, 2012. www.prohealth.com /library/showarticle.cfm?libid=16896 (accessed April 25, 2017).

Rivas, Anthony. "Drinking Coffee Can Lower Alzheimer's Risk By 20 Percent, All It Takes Is 3 Cups a Day." *Medical Daily,* November 26, 2014. www .medicaldaily.com/drinking-coffee-can-lower-alzheimers-risk-20-all-it-takes -3-cups-day-312410 (accessed April 25, 2017).

Sample, Ian. "Coffee May Boost Brain's Ability to Store Long-Term Memories, Study Claims." *Guardian,* January 12, 2014. www.theguardian.com/science /2014/jan/12/coffee-boost-brain-long-term-memories (accessed April 25, 2017).

Sarich, Christina. "Cilantro and Chlorella Can Remove 80 Percent of Heavy Metals from the Body Within 42 Days." *Natural Society,* July 7, 2014. http://naturalsociety.com/proper-heavy-metal-chelation-cilantro-chlorella (accessed April 25, 2017).

Sauer, Alissa. "The Effects of Medical Marijuana on Alzheimer's Treatment." Alzheimers.net, June 15, 2015. www.alzheimers.net/6-15-15-effects-of-medical-marijuana-on-alzheimers/ (accessed April 25, 2017).

Stan. "Laughter Could Improve Memory According to Scientists." IHeartIntelligence.com, August 28, 2014. http://iheartintelligence.com/2014/08/28/laughter-increases-memory-abilities/ (accessed April 25, 2017).

University of Eastern Finland. "Several Forms of Vitamin E Protect Against Memory Disorders, Study Says." *Science Daily,* January 7, 2014. www.sciencedaily.com/releases/2014/01/140107102640.htm (accessed April 25, 2017).

University Health News. "Can a Magnesium Supplement Reverse Memory Loss in Alzheimer's Patients?" March 17, 2017. http://universityhealthnews.com/daily/memory/the-best-magnesium-supplement-for-reversing-memory-loss-in-alzheimers/ (accessed May 2, 2017).

University of Tsukuba. "Active Body, Active Mind: The Secret to a Younger Brain May Lie in Exercising Your Body." October 28, 2015. www.tsukuba.ac.jp/en/research-list/p201510281125 (accessed April 25, 2017).

Worldhealth.net. "Diabetes: Alzheimer's Link." July 15, 2015. www.worldhealth.net/news/diabetes-alzheimers-link/ (accessed April 25, 2017).

Worldhealth.net. "Resveratrol Helps Memory." September 10, 2014. www.worldhealth.net/news/resveratrol-helps-memory/ (accessed April 25, 2017).

Worldhealth.net. "Vitamin E Slows Functional Decline." January 16, 2014. www.worldhealth.net/news/vitamin-e-slows-functional-decline/ (accessed April 25, 2017).

Wright, Jonathan V. "Lithium: The Misunderstood Mineral Part 1." Tahoma Clinic, May 4, 2010. http://tahomaclinic.com/2010/05/lithium-the-misunderstood-mineral-part-1/ (accessed April 25, 2017).

8

THE MIND-BODY CONNECTION

My body, mind, and spirit are a healing team.

LOUISE HAY

An old man was dealing with a cancer called lymphosarcoma. He visited the doctors frequently, but the cancer was quite advanced, and the news was grave. All the treatments had failed, and his body was full of large tumors. Fluid filled his chest cavity, making it necessary to drain it daily in order for him to breathe. He had no hope of recovery. However, he didn't want to give up, so he begged his doctor to put him on a new drug that could treat the cancer. Since he didn't meet the criteria for the trial of the drug, his requests were denied.

> The body's ability to heal is far greater than they have ever permitted you to believe.

Nothing, however, would stop the old man from persevering and getting the drug that he knew would cure him. After begging enough, the doctor finally gave in and gave him the injection of the drug. In reality, it was just an injection of water that the doctor had given in order to get him to stop begging. Two days later, the doctor was shocked to see that his patient was up and moving around like he hadn't done in months. Upon exam, the doctor found that the tumors had deteriorated drastically. Within ten days, the tumors had disappeared and the patient went home cancer free.

Soon, the medical journals reported that the drug that was the old man's medical cure was not effective. This caused the man great distress, and his tumors returned. His doctor was shocked by this change, and he decided to lift his patient's spirits once more by claiming that there was just one bad batch of the drug and that he had a good batch that he could give him. He injected his patient with water, and again the tumors disappeared. A while later, the man again heard reports of his miracle drug being worthless and his spirits fell, his cancer returned, and he died within two days.

The old man's belief that he would be healed by this drug ultimately cured him of his disease, even if the actual drug was not proven to work well. His mind was powerful enough to heal his body.

Another story that I find interesting comes from the South. Here, a midwife delivered three babies on Friday the thirteenth. Due to the date, the midwife proclaimed that these girls were hexed. The first girl born would die before her sixteenth birthday, the second before her twenty-first, and the third before her twenty-third. Sure enough, her predictions came true. The first two girls died a day before the birthdays they were not supposed to live to. The third girl went to the hospital the day before her twenty-third birthday with shortness of breath. She died a day short of her twenty-third birthday. Since all had believed the midwife's grave prediction, they sealed their fate to die young.

It is interesting how the mind can control our health and our well-being. We hear stories all the time about how people are miraculously healed. Is this due to a higher power or due to how we think and believe? The mind has a strong connection to our bodies and our overall health. Let's look at a few more examples of the mind controlling health.

It is said that a group of women were stricken blind after having to witness the torture and murders of people who were close to them. When they were examined, there was nothing physically wrong with their eyes that could explain the blindness. Seeing such gruesome events had made them not want to see, essentially making them blind.

Looking at another psychologically induced case of illness, we come across a woman with multiple personalities. While the condition should be completely psychological, there were some physical attributes that followed her personalities. One of her personalities had diabetes, while the other did not. When she was in her one personality, she would have high blood sugar and all the classic signs of diabetes. When she was the other personality, she had normal blood sugars and no signs of diabetes.

> **The human body possesses a profound and powerful regenerative capacity.**

A Greek war veteran was living in the United States when he was diagnosed with terminal lung cancer. While he was offered treatments, the doctors had very little hope of him surviving it. The man decided that he wanted to move back to his home country, where he could be near friends and family and be buried in the family cemetery. As time went on, instead of feeling worse, he actually started to feel better. He was relaxed and enjoyed his time with friends and family. Twenty-five years after his diagnosis, he went back to the United States to talk to his doctors about what had occurred, but none of them were still alive. The man ended up living to be 102 years old.

A final story I would like to share with you involves a young woman who was in the last stages of lymphoma. She felt herself being called to the other side. As she watched her loved ones below, she was given a choice. She could either stay in the light, or she could go back to her loved ones. She really didn't want to go back to a painful existence, but she was assured that if she did return to her life, the cancer would be cured. Believing this, she returned to her body, and to the astonishment of her doctors, went into spontaneous remission several days later.

The human body possesses a profound and powerful regenerative capacity. Time and again, serious diseases are suddenly and irrevocably reversed, much to the amazement of treating physicians. These extraordinary healings demonstrate the immense power of the body's ability to regenerate itself. The traditional medical systems of China, India, and Tibet are all based on the observation that the body will heal itself when it is brought back into balance. We should therefore do whatever is necessary to bring the body into healing balance. We should become aware of the power of this healing capacity.

Anecdotal evidence of seemingly anomalous miracle cures and faith healings have been reported throughout history. Psychologists have assembled empirical evidence pointing to the role of the mind and belief in achieving these effects for which there has been no scientific explanation. Recent research, however, has created an unprecedented bridge between the mind and the body. Experimental research demonstrates that we are just as capable of making ourselves sick, as making ourselves well!

Deepak Chopra in his SynchroDestiny teachings refers to a tribe in Australian Aboriginal culture that believes that if a stick is pointed at a person, they will soon get sick and eventually die. Time and again, a dispute in the tribe has proved this to be true. How do we explain that just pointing a stick at someone can cause death? It is of course the mind-body connection, or our belief system. We have all heard of miracle cures where someone was about to undergo an operation for a massive tumor, but a prayer group prayed for the person night and day, and when the doctors took a final CAT scan before performing the surgery, the tumor was completely gone. What these two examples illustrate is that the mind is far more powerful in healing the body than we have thought. You can use your mind to promote healing and even slow the aging process by reducing inflammation and cortisol production and increasing the production of life-enhancing hormones.

Dr. Lissa Rankin in her book *Mind over Medicine,* writes about the fact that what she had learned in medical school was missing something very important. This important lesson is the recognition of the body's innate ability to self-repair and how we can control this self-healing mechanism with the mind.

Now that we understand that mind-body medicine has a huge influence on the way we interpret illness and treat disease, it is time for us to use the concepts behind it to promote health and healing in our own lives.

In this chapter, we will examine the factors and the effects of the mind-body connection, how we can encourage the body's ability to heal, and what supplements and lifestyle modifications we can use that will assist in this endeavor.

THE HEALING POWER OF WATER

During the 1990s, Dr. Masaru Emoto noticed a connection between positive and negative energy when it came to water. Going further, he wanted to see if sending positive as opposed to negative energy at water would change the way its molecular arrangement played out.

With this in mind, Dr. Emoto used different sources of positive and negative energy and directed them at water. In his experiment, he used praise, soothing music, and even prayer to see how they affected water. Under a powerful microscope, he recorded the arrangement of molecules that went from total disarray to a beautiful, snowflakelike arrangement. It is apparent that the water was responding to the words aimed at it!

Now, let's think about this: the human body is made up of over 60 percent water. If we were to do the same things to our body that Dr. Emoto did to water, what would the effects be? Having positive energy aimed at the way we think about and treat our bodies could have significant healing impacts upon the progression of disease. Knowing this, why don't we surround ourselves with positive energy?

LONELINESS, AGING, AND DEPRESSION

It is no secret that there has been a disturbing epidemic when it comes to people who feel lonely and depressed. Why is this and how can we change this? If we look back to even just twenty years ago, depression wasn't as much of a problem as it is today.

Societal pressures have made it so that people believe that they are not as good as they need to be. Media and other outlets have fed us the message in subtle ways for years. Our minds believe what they are being told, thus affecting our overall health and mental well-being. Learning to avoid these negative viewpoints that are prevalent in our society can be one of the first steps in healing our symptoms of loneliness and depression.

Take a moment and think about the messages that you have been telling yourself. Are you comparing yourself to others who seem to have it all together? Do you wish that you were good enough to have the perfect life, an adoring spouse, and the ability to do as you please? These may be the messages that are ultimately affecting your health. You are basing your mental health and well-being on societal standards, not what you want for your life.

If you wish to beat loneliness and depression, then it's time for you to change your thoughts and your attitudes toward yourself. You are unique and nothing can change that. Don't let society determine what you should be and what you should feel. Sneak positivity into your life and begin to see the life-changing effects it can give you!

YOUR GUT AS A "SECOND BRAIN"

In his book *The Second Brain: A Groundbreaking New Understanding of Nervous Disorders of the Stomach and Intestines,* Dr. Michael Gershon has made some startling discoveries. He has devoted his career to understanding the human bowel as well as the stomach, esophagus, small intestines, and colon. His thirty years of research have led to an extraordinary rediscovery that nerve cells in the gut act as a brain. This "second brain" can also affect our emotions.

> **What you eat can actually affect the way you feel.**

Treating your digestive system well will help in the mission to combat negativity in your life. We often eat when we feel depressed or down. More often than not, that food isn't life-sustaining but comforting. Be aware of how your mental and emotional well-being can affect your dietary choices, and vice versa.

Yes, we eat based upon emotions, but according to Dr. Gershon, there is also a neurological feedback between the brain and the stomach. The enteric nervous system makes it possible for the brain to feel the effects of what is going on with the stomach, and vice versa. When we experience emotions such as anger and fear, we can feel that in our stomach as well as in our brain. How is this so? Well, the vagus nerve relays messages from our stomach to our brain. They call this reaction "the second brain." So, don't discount your gut feelings!

Depression, Stress, and Aging

Knowing that the stomach is connected to the brain, it is natural that emotions such as depression and stress can affect us both mentally and physically. It has also been proven that stress and depression can accelerate the aging process.

With such a strong connection and communication between these two organs, it is important to keep your gut healthy to combat depression, inflammation, and aging.

LONELINESS CAN BE DANGEROUS TO YOUR OVERALL WELL-BEING

We have all experienced points in our lives where we feel lonely. No one is around for you to talk to and you just feel down on yourself. You might take this as a passing phase. For some, it is. For others, it's a chronic state that can affect total mental and physical well-being. Scientists have discovered that chronic loneliness is even unhealthier than obesity. While obesity affects the circulatory system, loneliness can affect the blood pressure, and lead to depression and other chronic health problems.

Loneliness can lead to more serious physical health problems.

Loneliness can affect anyone, but when it is found in older adults, the health consequences are more detrimental. Having a strong connection with friends and family in old age can improve loneliness and lead to a longer life. Those who experience loneliness, around 60 million Americans, run an almost 14 percent greater risk of premature death.

HOW SPIRITUALITY CAN INCREASE YOUR HAPPINESS

Spirituality can help you feel a greater sense of positive well-being. Having a connection to your spirit or your religion can help you feel happier and more energetic. People who feel more spiritual tend to hold grudges less, are more grateful for what they have, and overall, feel more at peace with life.

Experiencing spirituality can help you feel much better about your life and the circumstances you may face. People often associate spirituality as a connection to a higher being, nature, or to oneself. When you feel more spiritual, you feel more hopeful and at peace with your own life.

Spirituality Can Affect Health

It has been discovered that having faith and being spiritual will increase a person's chances of recovering from severe illness. Those who believe that there is a higher power with the ability to heal are more likely to show signs of improvement. Even for those who don't believe in a higher power, the faith that healing can happen and being positive about the outcome will increase the chances of healing.

Elements of Spirituality

The elements of spirituality can help a person feel better on a daily basis. Having faith, hope, forgiveness, love, and support, all help influence a person's mental well-being. For some, prayer is a great way to share their anxieties and hurts with a higher power. Those who are prayed for feel more loved and cherished than those who do not receive prayer.

Connecting with Nature

Spending time in nature is a great way to get yourself centered and help release stress and anxiety. Taking a walk and enjoying the beauty of nature can ease your tension and help you focus your energy on positive thinking. For those who take nature walks often, they find that they get sick less often and overall feel a better sense of well-being. Having frequent contact with nature can help improve mood and increase your chances of living.

Gratitude Practice

Being grateful for what we have in life adds more positivity to it. Try showing your gratitude for what you have rather than complaining about what you don't have. If you realize how fortunate you are right now, your overall mind-set will change, helping to improve your mind and body connection. People who are more grateful for what they have actually are healthier and live longer. So, the next time you think about how hard you have it, think about all the wonderful things that you have in your life! We'll talk about gratitude in more detail in a later chapter.

Meditation

Meditation is a great way to ease stress and anxiety. By taking your mind off your problems and stresses, you are focusing on your personal well-being. Take some time each day to pursue some sort of meditation. For some, this can be found in prayer, while for others, this can be spent in nature, marveling at the wonders of all that is natural!

Having a Purpose

Those who have a purpose to their lives find that they feel more positive and are able to cope with stress much better than those who deal with depression. Spirituality helps you find that purpose. Focusing your energy toward a positive aspect of your life will help relieve stress and depression.

If you can't find the purpose of your life, don't worry, I'll teach you how to give a meaningful purpose to your life in chapter 16.

Socialization with Like-Minded People

Having people around you who share the same thoughts and values can have a huge effect on your overall well-being. The people who spend time with loved ones, go to church, or find a sporting event to participate in, will be less likely to succumb to depression and loneliness. Figure out what you enjoy, and spend some time with people who enjoy the same things.

Practice Loving Kindness

Showing people that you care for them will not only boost their spirits, but it will boost yours as well. Take some time to do good for others and you will feel good in return. It is proven that if you feel good about doing something, you are less likely to feel depressed or lonely.

SUPPLEMENTS

If you are naturally prone to feelings of loneliness and depression, there are supplements that you can take to help ease these symptoms. Many people will go to the doctor and get prescribed antidepressants, but the truth is, an over-the-counter supplement can actually do just as much good as a prescription. The influences of these supplements helped many who deal with severe depression and loneliness.

Probiotics

Using probiotics has been proven to show similar effects as taking an antidepressant. The probiotics alter your brain functions in ways that help to alleviate the feelings of anxiety and depression. When eating products such as yogurt and other fermented foods, the areas of the brain that are linked to emotion are less likely to respond drastically to extreme emotions.

Keeping your intestinal flora balanced with probiotics will help your mental and physical health. Make sure that your diet is consistent with helping healthy probiotics live in your system.

GABA

As I've already mentioned, gama-aminobutyric acid, or GABA, is a powerful amino acid that affects the brain. This amino acid helps to induce sleep and control excitement and motor control. Another great thing about GABA is that it can be used to help treat anxiety and depression.

GABA supplements can be used to ease symptoms of extreme stress and anxiety. This helps calm the nervous and digestive systems. Symptoms of depression and anxiety are due to miscommunications caused by toxins we receive from our diet and environment. GABA helps to restore these connections better than an antidepressant.

The benefits of GABA don't end with helping depression and anxiety. The supplements have also been proven to help alleviate stress, induce calmness, and boost your immune system. You can achieve these benefits with a supplement or by eating foods high in GABA such as nuts and whole grains.

L-Theanine

L-theanine is a supplement that is extracted from tea and is believed to help aid focus, sleep, and boost the immune system. Studies have also shown that it helps produce dopamine, a hormone that helps boost feelings of well-being. Like GABA, L-theanine has been shown to alleviate symptoms of stress, anxiety, and depression. It can also increase concentration!

The use of L-theanine has been linked to better sleep, feeling calmer, and being able to focus better. This is a great alternative to using caffeine and antidepressants!

SAMe

SAMe is a supplement that has been proven to relieve stress and depression better than tricyclic antidepressants. While it isn't highly publicized in the medical field, the use of SAMe has the same effects as many of the prescription antidepressants with fewer side effects. It also helps alleviate symptoms of depression sooner than antidepressants.

The use of supplements can help you if you do experience the symptoms of depression. While trying to handle the problem in as natural a way as possible is best, dietary supplements can be beneficial if natural treatments do not work.

POINTS TO REMEMBER

A study of food as medicine is not complete without the understanding that the mind and the body have a strong connection. Emotions can affect the mind and body; stress and anxiety can actually age you more quickly, and having a positive outlook on life can help decrease these negative effects. This was illustrated through Dr. Emoto's study of how energies affect the molecular arrangement of water. Knowing that positivity leads to longevity and wellness provides ways to help boost mood and outlook on life.

Spirituality, a connection to nature, and being around people with similar interests have proven to help decrease loneliness and depression. Having something that helps you focus on the positive aspects of your life can greatly decrease feelings of loneliness and depression. Also, there are supplements out there that will help you to feel less depressed if natural methods do not work out like you hoped they would.

The mind is a powerful organ that can affect the body in more ways than you can understand. By supporting it and being positive, you are one step closer to overall health and well-being.

People suffer with loneliness and depression on a daily basis. However, many people are not aware of the effects that stress, loneliness, and depression can have on their overall health. By finding ways to boost mood and alleviate these harmful emotions, you will not only feel better mentally, but you will also feel better physically. Try finding things you enjoy and add positivity to your life. It will not only help your mood, it will also help your overall health! Your mind has a strong connection with your body, so treat them both right!

REFERENCES FOR CHAPTER 8

Amazing Green Tea. "Theanine Health Benefits: More Than a Relaxant." www .amazing-green-tea.com/theanine-health-benefits.html (accessed May 2, 2017).

European Society of Cardiology. "Symptoms of Depression Causally Linked to Coronary Heart Disease, Not to Stroke." *Science Daily,* February 3, 2013. www.sciencedaily.com/releases/2014/02/140203191727.htm (accessed May 2, 2017).

Johnson, T. D. "SAMe." *LifeExtension,* April, 2007. http://www.lifeextension .com/Magazine/2007/4/report_same/Page-01 (accessed May 2, 2017).

Gupta, Sanjay. "Why You Should Treat Loneliness as a Chronic Illness." *Everyday Health,* August 4, 2015. www.everydayhealth.com/news/loneliness -can-really-hurt-you/ (accessed May 2, 2017).

Hadhazy, Adam. "Think Twice: How the Gut's 'Second Brain' Influences Mood and Well-Being." *Scientific American,* February 12, 2010. www .scientificamerican.com/article/gut-second-brain/ (accessed May 2, 2017).

Khazan, Olga. "How Walking in Nature Prevents Depression." *Atlantic,* June 30, 2015. www.theatlantic.com/health/archive/2015/06/how-walking-in -nature-prevents-depression/397172/ (accessed May 2, 2017).

Kurtus, Ron. "Importance of Spiritual Health in Life." Ron Kurtus' School for Champions, February 17, 2000. www.school-for-champions.com/life /importance_of_spiritual_health.htm (accessed May 2, 2017).

Ling, Kristi. "A Simple Secret for Living to 100 and Beyond." *HuffPost,* July 19, 2013. www.huffingtonpost.com/kristi-blicharski/secrets-to-living-longer _b_3606631.html (accessed May 2, 2017).

Mercola, Joseph. "Are Probiotics the New Prozac?" *Mercola,* July 25, 2013. http://articles.mercola.com/sites/articles/archive/2013/07/25/probiotics -new-prozac.aspx (accessed May 2, 2017).

Sample, Ian. "Loneliness Twice as Unhealthy as Obesity for Older People, Study Finds." *Guardian,* February 16, 2014. www.theguardian.com/science/2014 /feb/16/loneliness-twice-as-unhealthy-as-obesity-older-people (accessed May 2, 2017).

Umeå University. "Depression and Chronic Stress Accelerates Aging." *Science Daily,* November 9, 2011. www.sciencedaily.com/releases/2011/11/111109093729 .htm (accessed May 2, 2017).

University of Chicago. "Loneliness Is a Major Health Risk for Older Adults." *Science Daily,* February 16, 2014. www.sciencedaily.com /releases/2014/02/140216151411.htm (accessed May 2, 2017).

University of Maryland Medical Center. "Spirituality." http://umm.edu/health /medical/altmed/treatment/spirituality (accessed May 2, 2017).

University of Minnesota. "Everyday Access to Nature Improves Quality of Life in Older Adults." *Science Daily,* July 9, 2015. www.sciencedaily.com /releases/2015/07/150709180208.htm (accessed May 2, 2017).

Veterinärmedizinische Universität Wien. "The Long and the Short of Telomeres: Loneliness Impacts DNA Repair, Parrot Study Shows." *Science Daily,* April 4, 2014. www.sciencedaily.com/releases/2014/04/140404221746.htm (accessed May 2, 2017).

Wright, Carolanne. "How Microbes in the Gut Influence Anxiety, Depression." *Natural News,* May 5, 2014. www.naturalnews.com/044988_gut_bacteria _probiotics_microbiota.html (accessed May 2, 2017).

PART 3

The Search for a Solution

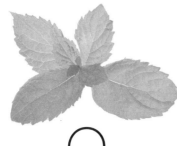

9

SUPPLEMENTING YOUR EVERYDAY NEEDS

Most people don't realize it, but when armed with the right knowledge and natural therapies, they are more capable of healing their bodies than they ever imagined.

JULIAN WHITAKER, M.D.,
THE WHITAKER WELLNESS INSTITUTE

Mary came to my office complaining of restless leg syndrome. She asked her doctor about vitamins. He replied that he doesn't believe in vitamins because you can get all the nutrients from your food. I explained to her that I lived in a farming community, and when the crops are harvested the soil is sandy, lacking any nutrients unless it is augmented. Also, studies have shown that the same type of carrots picked from two different places varied greatly in the amount of beta-carotene and vitamin A, so relying on diet alone in this age of pesticides and depleted soils is not the greatest idea.

I told her about pycnogenol and the studies that were done on restless leg syndrome. She began taking it and reported back in a month that her restless leg syndrome was gone.

Another example of how supplements can be used to heal is the story of Barbara. She was referred to me by her physician. She complained of chronic knee pain and had arthritis in both knees. She claimed it was bone on bone. She was seriously contemplating knee replacement surgery.

I informed her that there were a lot of studies on hyaluronic acid and knee osteoarthritis. In fact doctors even give injections of this every six months. This is made from rooster comb and helps lubricate and cushion the knee.

Barbara began taking 200 mg twice per day and noticed almost immediately that all her knee pain was gone. To this day she has not had surgery, but continues to take the supplement daily.

The twenty-first century is ushering in a new era of nutritional science. Western medicine has traditionally been focused on using drugs to relieve symptoms and to fight diseases but new research is showing that proper nutrition and a healthy lifestyle can help fight almost all kinds of diseases. Supplements can provide you with the kind of wholesome nutrition that can reduce the risk of getting age-related diseases such as heart disease, cancer, and dementia.

But that's not all. Some supplements might even be able to actually fight aging itself! New research is showing that nutrition might be the answer to not just slowing down aging but also possibly reversing it. The search for the fountain of youth is no longer a fairy tale.

Supplements can provide you with wholesome nutrition.

In this chapter, we will discuss this emerging research on anti-aging and also point you to certain "superstar" supplements that are not as popular in the mainstream media yet. But let's begin by talking about a key finding about telomeres and how they affect aging.

TELOMERES

Telomeres are a part of our DNA and new research on aging has shown that their length is directly related to aging. To understand how telomeres affect aging, first you need to understand what they are.

Every cell in the body has a nucleus, which holds the chromosomes. These chromosomes hold the genetic information related to our cells. When a cell divides, the chromosomes are replicated to make sure that the new cells also hold all the necessary genetic information. Each chromosome is made up of two arms of DNA. We've all heard about the DNA. These two arms hold all the information required for the building and functioning of the cells. The DNA holds this information in the form of bases. You don't need to know how these bases are made and how they hold the information. It is enough to understand that there are about 100 million information-holding bases in the DNA.

Now, the telomeres are found at the ends of each arm of DNA. They are like endcaps, keeping the DNA together during replication. The telomeres are made up of around 15,000 bases at the moment of conception of a new human being. Each time the cells replicate, the telomeres shorten a bit. The process of replication shortens the telomeres. If there were no telomeres, the DNA would be shortened and vital information would be lost and life would not be possible at all. So telomeres play a very important role in providing security to the DNA. When they reach the length of around 5,000 bases, the cells begin to die and eventually we die as well. This is the normal process of aging, leading to death.

Telomere shortening is a direct sign of aging.

It is important to note that this is not the only reason why we age. There are several processes taking place at the same time but telomere length is a direct indication of the age of a person. Mice and primates have much longer telomeres than humans but they don't live as long as we do. So telomere length is just one of many factors that affect aging.

In 1962, Leonard Hayflick gave the limit of 120 years as the maximum potential life-span for humans. This is known as the Hayflick limit and is based on the fact that around this time the cells can no longer replicate. In 1973, Alexey Olovnikov discovered that the telomeres shorten each time the cell divides because they cannot replicate completely.

Hence it was established that telomere shortening is a sign of aging. Then in 1984, Elizabeth Blackburn of the University of California–San

Francisco discovered that the enzyme telomerase has the ability to lengthen the telomere by synthesizing DNA from an RNA primer. She, along with her two colleagues, received the Nobel Prize in Physiology in 2009. This finding has become very important for anti-aging researchers, and some scientists believe that by using nutrition to lengthen telomeres, humans can achieve the life-span of up to 150 years!

Effects of Telomere Shortening

Telomere shortening has also been found to be related to age-related diseases such as heart disease, cancer, and dementia. Lawrence Honig of Columbia University conducted a study on 1,983 patients with a mean age of 78. The study followed the participants for 10 or more years. Of the participants, 190 developed dementia and it was found that telomere length was shorter in these cases than in those who did not get dementia.

Telomere shortening has also been linked to decreased immune response against infections, type 2 diabetes, atherosclerotic lesions, neurodegenerative diseases, testicular cancer, intestinal atrophy, and DNA damage. The rate at which telomeres shorten might also be able to indicate the risk of cancer.

Scientists from Northwestern University and Harvard have developed such a technique by studying the telomere length of patients who were eventually diagnosed with cancer. These patients had a high rate of telomere shortening, but 3 to 4 years before diagnoses, the shortening stopped. They found that cancer cells took over the telomeres and stopped their shortening in order to divide and replicate indefinitely. This could help diagnose cancer much quicker than the current methods.

Studies done in Denmark and at the University of Utah have also shown that shorter telomere length is linked to shorter life expectancy and higher risk of premature death.

Nutrition and Telomere Length

Nutrition is an important factor for telomere length and health. Telomeres get damaged more easily than DNA and an unhealthy telomere is just as bad as a short telomere. So both the quality and quantity are important and both are affected by nutrition. For example, healthy mothers who get proper nutrition give birth to children with optimal telomere length and quality.

To understand how nutrition helps improve telomere health and length, you need to know about a process called methylation. This is the chemical process of donating a methyl group (a CH_3 molecule) to the genetic material of the telomere. This process marks the telomeres for proper functioning and it is a very important process for proper health and functioning of the telomeres.

In order to achieve this methylation, the body needs methyl donors. One important methyl donor is S-Adenosyl-L-methionine (SAMe). SAMe is a very important metabolite and it requires nutrients such as methionine, MSM sulfur, choline, and trimethylglycine. These form the building blocks of SAMe along with vitamin B_{12}, B_6, and folic acid. You can get SAMe as a supplement but it is better to let the body build it naturally using the building-block nutrients.

You can get all of these nutrients through a good multivitamin, along with some sulfur-rich protein such as whey protein, eggs, cottage cheese, dairy, red meat, chicken, legumes, duck, nuts, and seeds. Eggs contain more choline than any other food source.

One way to know if you are short on methyl donors is to monitor your mood. The brain requires methyl donors to stay healthy and a bad mood is a sign of shortage of methyl donors. It can even lead to chronic depression. By taking multivitamins and proteins you can increase methyl donors in your body and you will see it as a change in your mood. If your brain has enough methyl donors then that means there are enough methyl donors for the healthy functioning of telomeres as well.

A study done on 586 women found that those who took multivitamins regularly had 5 percent longer telomeres. Another study found that men with higher folic acid levels had longer telomeres. Yet another study showed that both men and women who had low levels of folate also had shorter telomeres.

Minerals and antioxidants are also important nutritional elements for healthy telomeres. Antioxidants reduce the amount of free radicals, which can damage the telomeres. Magnesium is important for enzymes that help in DNA replication. A study found that magnesium deprivation causes rapid loss of telomere length. The adequate amount of magnesium is from 400 mg to 800 mg per day but sadly there is a lot of magnesium deficiency in the American diet.

Zinc is another mineral that helps in DNA repair. Lack of zinc can lead to excessive breakage of DNA strands. The minimum amount of zinc you need is 15 mg per day with the maximum being 50 mg to 75 mg for women and men, respectively. Carnosine is an antioxidant that contains zinc and has been shown to reduce the rate of telomere depletion in human fibroblast cells and extend their longevity. It is also a good brain antioxidant.

Certain vitamins have also been known to help in maintaining telomere length. Vitamin C has been found to slow the loss of telomere length in human vascular endothelial cells. Vitamin D fights inflammation and supports telomere length. A study done on 2,100 female twins between the ages of 19 and 79 found that highest levels of vitamin D corresponded to the longest telomeres. The women with the shortest telomeres also had the lowest levels of vitamin D and the difference accounted for about 5 years of potential life-span.

Vitamin E, especially tocotrienols, has been shown to actually restore telomere length in human fibroblast cells. They also help in restoring damaged DNA and so this vitamin is a prime candidate for an anti-aging drug.

Factors Affecting Telomere Length

An unhealthy lifestyle that includes eating junk food, smoking, and sedentary habits can lead to shorter telomeres. Professor Dean Ornish of the University of California did a study on thirty-five men with prostate cancer. Ten of the men were told to change their lifestyle and go on a health kick. They ate vegetarian food and did regular exercise, meditation, and yoga to bust stress.

> **An unhealthy lifestyle increases the rate of telomere shortening. So basically you are growing old faster!**

After 5 years, the telomeres in these 10 men grew longer by 10 percent while in the remaining 25 they decreased by 3 percent. This is only a short pilot study and large randomized trials need to be conducted, but it looks like a healthy lifestyle and proper nutrition can actually turn back the clock on aging.

Obesity causes higher free-radical damage, and inflammation leads to higher telomere loss. Stress and infection can lead to inflammation and hence shorter telomeres. Inflammation also causes an increase in the cell turnover rate, which means the telomeres get shortened quickly. It's as if you are running out of life faster than others. DHA and vitamin D are great for fighting inflammation. A study done on 608 cardiovascular patients over a five-year period showed that those who had a higher intake of DHA/EPA had longer telomeres.

The gene signal that causes inflammation is known as NF-kappaB. Nutrients such as those found in fruits, vegetables, nuts, and whole grains can actually calm this signal and reduce inflammation. Other nutrients that preserve telomere length are quercetin, green tea catechins, grape-seed extract, curcumin, and resveratrol. Grape-seed extract and curcumin are especially beneficial because they help in generating longer telomeres.

Calorie restriction is another good way of lengthening telomeres. Eating excessively on a regular basis shortens telomeres. But calorie restriction activates the sirtuin 1 (sirt1) gene, which helps the body to maintain primary systems during food scarcity. This leads to preservation of longer telomeres. Resveratrol also activates the sirt1 gene.

Stress has also been found to be a contributing factor to shortened telomeres. A study done by Nobel Prize winner Elizabeth Blackburn in 2004, looked at the effect of stress on female caregivers. The ones who reported facing higher stress levels had shorter telomeres. The difference between women with the shortest telomeres and the longest telomeres was equivalent to one decade of aging! PTSD and childhood trauma have both been linked to shorter telomeres. The good news is that exercise has been found to be able to reverse the damage caused by stress. A study done on women with childhood trauma found that those who exercised vigorously had longer telomeres than the women who were abused as children but did not exercise.

High-intensity exercise is especially important in improving telomere health and length. Exercises like Peak 8, where you raise your heart rate to the anaerobic threshold with high intensity exercise for twenty to thirty seconds and then recover for ninety seconds and then repeat this cycle eight times, are much better than normal cardio exercises at improving telomere length. This type of short-burst, high-intensity exercise also produces the human growth hormone that helps in restoring damage to DNA.

SUPPLEMENTS

Now let's talk about a few supplements in particular and see how they can help us achieve a nutritional balance that will keep us healthy and may even delay aging and age-related diseases.

TA-65

TA-65 is the product name for the compound cycloastragenol, which is extracted from the Chinese herb astragalus. It was developed by Geron Corporation and sold to T.A. Sciences, who manufacture it as TA-65. It works by activating an enzyme called telomerase. This enzyme helps rebuild telomeres after cell division. It is active in reproductive cells and the telomere length of these cells does not shorten like other cells. Some researchers feel that by activating telomerase, telomere health and length can be improved.

The important thing to note about telomerase is that other researchers have found that high telomerase activity is related to cancer formation. The cancer cells activate telomerase, which restores telomere length and that in turn allows the cancer cells to divide uncontrollably.

There are studies done on both sides of this debate and the final conclusion is still to be made. For one thing, a lot of the studies have been done by T.A. Sciences and Geron Corporation, who have vested interests in the product. Their studies showed a decrease in the percentage of very short telomeres in mice but did not show an increase in the average telomere length.

Also, telomeres are just one of many factors in aging. Shorter telomeres are certainly a sign of aging but they are not the only factor, so lengthening your telomeres alone and doing nothing else won't necessarily make you live longer. That being said, improving telomere health through telomerase activation can be the right direction in the field of anti-aging and we need more large-scale neutral studies to be done on it.

The good news is that telomerase can be activated naturally as well.

You can activate telomerase enzyme by eating healthy, exercising, and meditating. Eat lots of fruit and vegetables, healthy fats, lean protein, and drink lots of water. Even simple exercise like a brisk thirty-minute walk can help reduce stress and activate telomerase in the body. Meditation too is good for busting stress. Along with a healthy lifestyle you can look into TA-65 as an additional supplement as long as you do some research and keep in mind that this new supplement still needs to pass the test of time to ensure it has no bad side effects.

Astaxanthin

We've already talked about astaxanthin in previous chapters. It is a remarkable natural antioxidant that is 6,000 times more powerful than vitamin C in terms of its antioxidant properties. It is a carotenoid that is naturally found in algae and the animals that eat those algae such as shrimps, lobsters, crabs, salmon, and flamingos. It gives these animals their red/pink color. Because of its unique structure it always remains an antioxidant and never becomes a pro-oxidant like some other antioxidants.

Astaxanthin is one supplement you must have in your diet.

Astaxanthin has a lot of beneficial properties. It protects the marine life from ultraviolet radiation of the sun; in the beginning researchers were looking to use it as a sunscreen. But now a lot more benefits have been discovered. Almost every part of your body can benefit from astaxanthin, including your skin, eyes, heart, kidneys, and brain.

Apart from its ability to absorb ultraviolet radiation, being an antioxidant means that it scavenges and neutralizes free radicals. It also provides mitochondrial protection, has anti-inflammatory properties, and protects from glycation. It also slows down age-related cognitive decline.

Here are the benefits of astaxanthin in more detail:

Relieves Pain and Inflammation: Astaxanthin has very good analgesic and anti-inflammatory properties. It works as well as some prescription pain medications and since it is completely natural it doesn't have side effects that some analgesics have, such as addiction, heartburn, and gastrointestinal bleeding. Astaxanthin blocks cyclooxygenase-2 (COX-2) enzyme, which is exactly what drugs like Celebrex do. It also suppresses nitric oxide (NO) serum levels, prostaglandin E2, interleukin 1B, tumor necrosis factor alpha (TNF-alpha), and C Reactive Protein (CRP). All of these factors are related to pain, inflammation, and fever.

Skin Protection: Astaxanthin can provide protection to the skin from the harmful UV rays, from within the skin. This means that sun-rays are absorbed and their beneficial effect of producing vitamin D is not diminished. Instead astaxanthin fights the free radicals that are introduced by the radiation. It has a large number of electrons to give to the free radicals and it doesn't break down to become a free radical itself. It can help keep the skin moist and prevent wrinkles, spots, and loss of elasticity.

Boosts Immune Function: Astaxanthin helps balance the immune system so that it remains active to fight against diseases, but doesn't become overactive and cause allergic reactions. It increases the number of white blood cells in the body. But at the same time it protects against damage to lymphocytes and neutrophils caused by overactive white blood cells. It works like antihistamine drugs such as Cetirizine.

Fights Age-Related Cognitive Decline: Astaxanthin is able to cross the blood-brain barrier and so is better at protecting the brain from free-radical damage than most other antioxidants. It fights the abnormal proteins such as amyloid beta, which causes neuro-degenerative diseases such as Alzheimer's and Parkinson's. It can also improve learning and lower age-related forgetfulness.

Fights Cancer: Astaxanthin along with other carotenoids lowers the risk of cancer of all kinds. It fights cancer at every stage of the disease. It protects DNA from oxidative damage and prevents cancer from starting. It improves the immune system that can destroy cancer cells during the early stages. It restricts the growth of cancer cells by reducing inflammation. It fights rapid cancer cell division and replication. It keeps the size of tumors small by restricting production of tissue-melting proteins by tumors.

Good for the Eyes: Astaxanthin has been found to be effective against eye diseases such as glaucoma, cataract, and age-related macular degeneration. Astaxanthin can reach your retina, which already has other carotenoids such as lutein and zeaxanthin. In studies done on patients with macular degeneration, a combination of carotenoids helped in improving visual acuity and contrast detection. The carotenoids they used were astaxanthin (4 mg/day), lutein (10 mg/day), and zeaxanthin (1 mg/day).

Good for the Cardiovascular System: Astaxanthin can lower blood pressure and hypertension. It can also help in maintaining lipid profiles, reducing triglyceride and cholesterol levels while boosting the beneficial HDL cholesterol. It can also help in improving mitochondrial energy delivery in the heart muscle, which helps the heart be more powerful and efficient. This comes in handy especially during a heart attack when the remaining muscles have to take over the job of the damaged muscles.

Reduces Diabetes: Astaxanthin also helps in lowering blood glucose level, improves insulin sensitivity, and reduces inflammation and damage from free radicals. All of this helps in fighting diabetes and the related disorder of obesity. It also preserves the ability of the pancreas to produce insulin. It helps in reducing the complications of diabetes such as cataract formation, diabetic retinopathy, and cardiovascular complications.

Fights Fatigue: Astaxanthin is used by many athletes because it helps them recover quickly from strenuous exercise. It has been found to provide immense endurance to salmon that swim upriver to lay their eggs. It helps in improving endurance, increasing energy levels, and increasing strength of the muscles.

All of these wonderful benefits can be yours if you include astaxanthin in your diet. One of the best sources of astaxanthin is wild-caught salmon. But diet alone might not be able to provide enough astaxanthin that is readily absorbed by the body. In order to increase its bioavailability you should take astaxanthin supplements that have natural astaxanthin along with phospholipids. Astaxanthin mixes poorly with water and is more readily soluble in oil or fat. Phospholipids act as emulsifying agents and thus increase absorption of astaxanthin by as much as twelve times. It's also a good idea to take astaxanthin supplement with a meal that has the most fat.

Nattokinase

Nattokinase is an enzyme that is found in a Japanese breakfast food called natto. Natto is made of soybeans that have been fermented using the *Bacillus subtilis* bacteria. These bacteria act on the soybeans to produce the nattokinase enzyme. Natto is a pungent cheeselike food with a nutty flavor and a slimy texture. It is eaten with rice, all over Japan, and has been known for thousands of years for its amazing health benefits. It has been used as a folk remedy for heart disease.

The nattokinase enzyme can break up and dissolve blood clots, lower blood pressure, and have a blood-thinning effect similar to aspirin and cardiovascular drugs. Nattokinase, being a natural substance, has a significant advantage over blood-thinning drugs because it can be used for longer periods without any serious side effects.

It was discovered by Dr. Hiroyuki Sumi, who had been testing different foods to find a natural thrombolytic agent to dissolve blood clots. He applied natto to a blood clot in a Petri dish at body temperature and in just eighteen hours the clot was completely dissolved. He named the enzyme nattokinase, which means "enzyme in natto."

Nattokinase can:

- Dissolve fibrins (the fibers that build up to form a clot)
- Dissolve existing blood clots
- Prevent blood clots from forming
- Support normal blood pressure
- Increase the production of plasmin, urokinase, and other blood clot dissolving agents that the body manufactures

Around seventeen studies have been done on nattokinase and two of them have been small human trials. A study done on twelve healthy Japanese men and women by Miyazaki Medical College, Oklahoma State University, and JCR Pharmaceuticals found that those who were given 7 ounces of natto before breakfast had the ability to dissolve clots twice as fast as the control group.

Their blood plasma sample was taken and an artificial clot was induced to see how fast it dissolved. The natto group also retained the ability to dissolve blood clots for eight hours longer than the control group.

In another study, a group of human volunteers with high blood pressure were given natto extract for four days. In four out of five volunteers the systolic blood pressure dropped from the average of 173.8 to 154.8 and the diastolic blood pressure from the average of 101 to 91.2.

You can prepare natto to eat as a food but if the taste is not for you, then you can get nattokinase as a supplement. Nattokinase is safe if used according to the recommended dosage. People with low blood pressure, blood-thinning problems, or those who already take blood thinners, have ulcers, or are recovering from surgery should not take nattokinase. It can leave you prone to bruising and might hinder the ability to stop bleeding, which are both common side effects of blood-thinning drugs, but the effect of nattokinase is not as pronounced as the drugs.

You should take nattokinase supplement if you have a cardiovascular disease and are looking for a safe alternative to the common aspirin-based drugs. Long flights can cause deep vein thrombosis and natto taken before or during a flight can help with this issue. In any situation where you would take a blood-thinning medicine, nattokinase can be used as an alternative that has fewer side effects, has a prolonged effect, and is much cheaper.

Vitamin D

Vitamin D is a supernutrient. It is more like a hormone than a vitamin. It can activate about 2,000 genes in the human body. Vitamin D also activates enzymes in the brain that help in nerve growth. It can protect neurons by boosting glutathione production. It also enhances the immune system and has anti-inflammatory properties.

Here are some of the benefits of vitamin D:

- Boosts cognitive function
- Keeps the brain healthy and protects it from neurodegeneration
- Low levels of vitamin D have been correlated with depression,

abdominal obesity, osteoarthritis, low testosterone levels, and pelvic floor disorders

• Reduces risk of diabetes

Vitamin D deficiency is very common because people don't get enough sun exposure anymore. This leads to the three deadly *D*'s in seniors: depression, dementia, and diabetes. The risk of all of these can be lowered by maintaining optimal levels of vitamin D in the body. This is supposed to be around 50 to 70 mg/ml.

Sun exposure is one of the best ways to get vitamin D. The UV radiation causes the body to produce vitamin D. You have to be careful to not get overexposure as that can lead to sunburn and even skin cancer. But our current lifestyle puts us more at risk for vitamin D deficiency than skin cancer. Tanning can also provide a similar reaction in the body. But if for some reason you can't get enough sun exposure, then vitamin D supplements are the way to go.

Remember to also take vitamin K2 if you are taking vitamin D, because K2 helps in avoiding the side effects of vitamin D toxicity. Vitamin D creates some proteins that need vitamin K2 to get activated. These proteins then help move calcium around the body, removing it from places it is not supposed to be, like the arteries, and carrying it to the places where it should be, like bones. These two vitamins taken together help to keep you happy, improve cognition, protect the brain, keep your bones strong, and improve heart health.

Pycnogenol

Pycnogenol comes from a French pine tree bark and contains flavonoids such as procyanidins and phenolic acids. These phytonutrients are very important for maintaining proper health. Pycnogenol has the ability to prevent oxidative stress, membrane damage, DNA damage, inflammation, and glycation.

It is a supplement that has a lot of benefits and close to zero side effects. It can help with diseases such as diabetes, diabetic retinopathy, asthma, menopause, impotence, osteoarthritis, deep vein thrombosis, and hypertension. It can have effects similar to nattokinase in terms of blood thinning. It also has antioxidant and anti-inflammatory properties.

In a study, a group of smokers were given either 500 mg of aspirin or

120 mg of pycnogenol and the amount of platelet clumping, which leads to blood clots, was measured. Pycnogenol had just as much effect as aspirin in reducing clumping. It is also known to boost production of nitrous oxide, which helps the arteries to stay open and relaxed, which in turn maintains a healthy blood pressure.

A double-blind, placebo-controlled trial was conducted on sixty kids between the ages of 6 and 18 with mild to moderate asthma. After three months, the kids who were on pycnogenol had better pulmonary function and reduced asthma symptoms along with reduced leukotrienes, a marker for inflammation. Studies on adults have shown similar results for asthma patients.

Pycnogenol works really well with and improves the effects of vitamin C. In a study, people suffering from the common cold were told to take pycnogenol, vitamin C, and zinc supplements and their colds resolved in just four days as compared to seven days for untreated common cold. They also suffered less from the symptoms of common cold like runny nose, congestion, sneezing, cough, and sore throat.

As already mentioned in chapter 5, pycnogenol fights the signs of aging because of its antioxidant and anti-inflammatory properties. It protects collagen and elastin and acts as an internal sunscreen. It also improves skin hydration and reduces skin pigmentation.

Pycnogenol can help with erectile dysfunction when combined with L-arginine. Because of its ability to improve blood flow it is a good idea to take this supplement before a long flight to prevent deep vein thrombosis. It has also been found that cancer patients going through chemotherapy find relief from side effects such as vomiting, diarrhea, and weight loss when they take pycnogenol.

Phosphatidylserine

Phosphatidylserine (PS) is a major phospholipid found in the brain. It is a constituent of cell membranes of the nerve cells. It helps in maintaining the fluidity of the nerve cells so that they can release the neurotransmitters acetylcholine and dopamine. The body manufactures PS on its own to keep us mentally acute, but as we grow older the production of PS drops. That's where PS supplements come in.

PS deficiency is linked to mental impairment, dementia including

Alzheimer's, depression, and Parkinson's disease. PS supplements can improve and even reverse symptoms of age-related cognitive decline.

It restocks brain cell membranes, it boosts production of nerve chemicals such as dopamine and serotonin, it lowers stress hormones, it stimulates nerve cell growth, and can possibly even generate new neural connections. It activates all brain centers especially the hypothalamus, the cortex, and the pituitary gland. In short, you can say that PS supplements can reverse aging of nerve cells.

A study was done on fifty-year-old men with dementia in which 300 mg of PS taken daily for 3 months was able to improve mental function. Another study with Alzheimer's patients found that even as little as 100 mg per day for 3 months helped in improving cognitive abilities.

People who suffer from normal loss in memory power caused by aging also experience improvements in their memory power upon taking 100 mg of PS daily for 12 weeks. Experts believe that 300 mg taken per day in three doses of 100 mg each is sufficient for those experiencing symptoms of age-related cognitive decline.

In healthy males, 800 mg of PS taken daily for ten days was reported to cause a reduction in stress response by the hypothalamus, the pituitary gland, and the adrenal glands. As a preemptive treatment, healthy young people can take 50 to 75 mg of PS per day to reduce cortisol response to stress, which will improve your overall health. PS can also activate the cells of the immune system and give it a boost.

PS used to be obtained from the brains of cows but there was a slight risk of mad cow disease. Now PS is obtained from soy lecithin by using an enzyme that converts the phosphatidycholine into phosphatidylserine. It can also be isolated from egg yolks using a similar process. When you buy PS supplements, make sure that it is phosphatidylserine and not phosphorylated serine, which doesn't have the same effects as PS. PS supplements aren't known to have any adverse side effects.

Glutathione

Glutathione is a molecule made up of cysteine, glycine, and glutamine. It is produced naturally in the body and is a very powerful element of the body's natural health mechanisms. It is the best antioxidant produced by the body.

It is the key to our detoxification system. And it also provides major support to the immune system.

Best of all, the body is able to recycle glutathione naturally so, technically, we should never run out of it. But the truth is that because of our current lifestyle, we are prone to so many toxins and so much stress that our glutathione levels deplete quickly. This leaves us vulnerable to all kinds of diseases.

A diet lacking in nutrients, thousands of toxins present everywhere around us, pollution, stress, trauma, infections, radiation, and aging are all causes for glutathione depletion in the body. The body is simply overwhelmed and we don't have enough glutathione to deal with everything.

Depleted levels of glutathione can lead to high oxidative stress, which can destroy our cells and lead to infections and even cancer. It can cause diseases such as chronic fatigue syndrome, heart disease, cancer, infections, autoimmune diseases, autism, Alzheimer's, diabetes, arthritis, Parkinson's, asthma, kidney problems, liver disease, dementia, and premature aging. Reduced glutathione levels also lead to reduced physical performance, increased recovery time, increased muscle damage, and reduced strength and stamina.

This is why we need to find ways to increase our levels of glutathione. One way to do it is by eating the right foods. Sulfur-rich foods such as garlic, onions, and cruciferous vegetables provide the building blocks for glutathione. Bioactive whey protein is also a good source of cysteine and other amino acids that build glutathione in the body. Avocado, walnuts, poultry, and egg yolks are other foods that help in providing the building blocks for glutathione.

Exercising is another way of boosting glutathione levels in the body. Aerobic exercise for thirty minutes a day can significantly boost your glutathione levels.

Lastly, you can take glutathione as a supplement. Glutathione supplements have been around for a long time but the common scientific consensus was that these oral supplements were good for nothing because the body digests proteins and breaks down the oral glutathione present in the supplements.

But new improvements in this technology have come up with better supplements such as L-glutathione, liposomal glutathione, and acetyl glutathione; all of these are highly bioavailable and the body can readily absorb glutathione from these supplements.

Along with this, you should also look for supplements that contain glutathione precursors, which help the body to manufacture more glutathione. Some of the precursors are N-acetylcysteine (NAC), alpha lipoic acid (ALA), selenium, magnesium, B vitamins, vitamin E, and milk thistle.

Turmeric

Turmeric is a spice that is pretty common in Southeast Asian and Indian cuisine. It contains curcumin, a natural anti-inflammatory substance that has been found to help with diseases such as Alzheimer's, skin diseases, ulcers, colitis, diabetes, high cholesterol, and it eases pain and inflammation caused by arthritis and osteoarthritis. It also acts as an antioxidant. Curcumin has also been known to fight cancer and it stops the growth of certain tumors.

You can get turmeric as a spice and use it in your food or you can eat Indian or Southeast Asian cuisine, which contains turmeric in curry. You can also take curcumin supplements.

Longvida is one curcumin supplement that is highly bioavailable. It helps curcumin reach the brain where it can fight inflammation and can even break down amyloid beta plaques. There aren't any major side effects of curcumin and it is pretty safe to take as a supplement.

Resveratrol

Resveratrol is a polyphenol found in red grape skins and other plants like berries, peanuts, and dark chocolate. It is a great antioxidant because of the polyphenolic structure. It is good at fighting free-radical damage in the body and also in the brain. It has been known to prevent amyloid beta plaque buildup in the brain, which is the main cause of Alzheimer's. It also has a similar effect as nattokinase in terms of improving blood flow and dissolving clots.

This makes it a good supplement for those who suffer from heart disease. Some studies have also found that resveratrol can slow cancer growth. It can also prevent insulin resistance and hence prevent diabetes. It has an effect similar to that of calorie restriction and is touted as an anti-aging supplement. It also fights obesity by activating the sirt1 gene.

There aren't any significant side effects as it comes from natural sources. But because of its blood-thinning properties it should not be mixed with blood-thinning drugs. While buying resveratrol supplements make sure that it is extracted from natural sources.

POINTS TO REMEMBER

Telomeres, endcaps of DNA, are a sure marker for aging. As the cells divide, the telomeres protect the DNA information from being lost but in turn they themselves get shorter. The shorter the telomeres, the older the person is, and once the telomeres become too short, the cells can't divide properly and the person dies. This finding has been an important milestone in the field of anti-aging and the researchers even received a Nobel Prize when they found that telomerase enzyme can help restore telomere length.

Telomere shortening is a natural process but it can be hastened by lifestyle, diet, stress, and environmental factors. The good news is that telomere length can be maintained and even recovered with proper nutrition and lifestyle. If this information is not the key to the fountain of youth, it is certainly a big step in the right direction.

In order to maintain proper nutrition, we need to supplement our diet with certain key supplements. Multivitamins and minerals are important but there are also certain supplements that aren't that well known outside natural medicine circles because of lack of large studies, but they provide some tremendous health benefits.

Astaxanthin, nattokinase, pycnogenol, glutathione, resveratrol, phosphatidylserine, vitamin D, and curcumin are these supersupplements that should surely be a part of your diet.

REFERENCES FOR CHAPTER 9

Cohen, Suzy. "5 Reasons to Take Astaxanthin Every Day." *HuffPost,* February 28, 2013. www.huffingtonpost.com/entry/astaxanthin_b_2750910.html?section =india (accessed April 25, 2017).

Collins, Danica. "Dissolve Blood Clots with Nattokinase." Underground Health Reporter. http://undergroundhealthreporter.com/dissolve-blood-clots-with -nattokinase/ (accessed April 25, 2017).

Eliaz, Issac. "Telomeres: The New Key to Anti-Aging." *Easy Health Options.* http://easyhealthoptions.com/telomeres-the-new-key-to-anti-aging/ (accessed April 25, 2017).

GSHGold. "Glutathione Benefits." Gshgold.com/glutathione-benefits/ (accessed May 2, 2017).

Hawkins, Liam. "Astaxanthin Provides Broad Spectrum Protection." *Life Extension Magazine,* April, 2013. www.lifeextension.com/Magazine/2013/4/Astaxanthin -Provides-Broad-Spectrum-Protection/Page-01 (accessed May 9, 2017).

Health Freedom Alliance. "Regeneration of Brain Stem-Cell Linked with Turmeric Compound." March 27, 2016. www.healthfreedoms.org/regeneration-of -brain-stem-cell-linked-with-turmeric-compound/ (accessed April 25, 2017).

Herbwisdom.com. "Pycnogenol." www.herbwisdom.com/herb-pycnogenol.html (accessed April 25, 2017).

Heyes, J. D. "Your Depression May Be Due to Vitamin D Deficiency." *Natural News,* March 26, 2013. www.naturalnews.com/039643_depression_vitamin _D_deficiency.html (accessed April 25, 2017).

Hyman, Mark. "Glutathione: The Mother of All Antioxidants." *HuffPost,* June 10, 2010. www.huffingtonpost.com/entry/glutathione-the-mother -of_b_530494.html?section=india (accessed May 9, 2017).

James, Andy. "What Is Nattokinase and What Are Its Health Benefits." *Nattokinase Heart Health,* June 12, 2013. http://nattokinasehearthealth .com/20/what-is-nattokinase-and-health-benefits/ (accessed April 25, 2017).

Jockers, David. "Supercharge Your Brain with Sunshine." *Natural News,* March 26, 2013. www.naturalnews.com/039642_sunshine_cognitive_function_vitamin _D.html (accessed April 25, 2017).

Katie (Wellness Mama). "The Master Antioxidant: Glutathione." Wellnessmama .com, February 28, 2017. https://wellnessmama.com/37260/glutathione -benefits/ (accessed April 25, 2017)

Mercola, Joseph. "Astaxanthin: Nature's Most Powerful Antioxidant." *Mercola,* February 10, 2013. http://articles.mercola.com/sites/articles /archive/2013/02/10/cysewki-discloses-astaxanthin-benefits.aspx (accessed April 25, 2017).

———. "Discover How the Legendary Benefits of the Japanese Food 'Natto' Make for a Healthy Heart and Strong Bones." *Mercola.* www.mercola.com /Downloads/bonus/discover-the-benefits-of-natto/report.aspx (accessed April 25, 2017).

———. "Vitamin D for Depression, Dementia, and Diabetes," *Mercola,* August 21, 2014. http://articles.mercola.com/sites/articles/archive/2014/08/21/vitamin -d-depression-dementia.aspx (accessed April 25, 2017).

Mullan, Nancy. "One of the Most Promising Anti-Aging Breakthroughs I've Ever Seen." Nancy Mullan, MD. *Genetics Based Medicine,* February 2, 2013.

https://chronicdiseaserecovery.wordpress.com/2013/02/02/one-of-the-most
-promising-anti-aging-breakthroughs-ive-ever-seen/ (accessed April 25, 2017).

Richards, Byron J. "Nutrition Makes Anti-Aging Possible: Secrets of Your
Telomeres." *Byron J. Richards Wellness Resources,* May 21, 2013. www
.wellnessresources.com/health/articles/how_nutrition_makes_anti-aging
_possible_secrets_of_your_telomeres/ (accessed April 25, 2017).

Roberts, Michelle. "Health Kick 'Reverses Cell Aging.'" *BBC News,* September
16, 2013. www.bbc.com/news/health-24111357 (accessed April 25, 2017).

Sahelian, Ray. "Pycnogenol Supplement Benefits and Side Effects, Review of
Research Trials." February 1, 2016. www.raysahelian.com/pycnogenol.html
(accessed April 25, 2017).

Sarto, Janet. "Pycnogenol: Multi-Modal Defense Against Aging." *Life Extension
Magazine,* August, 2012.

SmartPublications. "Nattokinase: Powerful Enzyme Prevents Heart Attack
and Stroke." www.smart-publications.com/articles/nattokinase-powerful
-enzyme-prevents-heart-attack-and-stroke (accessed April 25, 2017).

Whitaker, Julian. "6 Surprising Benefits of Vitamin D." Dr. Whitaker, February 25,
2014. www.drwhitaker.com/6-surprising-benefits-of-vitamin-d (accessed
April 25, 2017).

———. "Benefits of Pycnogenol." Dr. Whitaker, July 18, 2014. www.drwhitaker
.com/benefits-of-pycnogenol/ (accessed April 25, 2017).

Wong, Cathy. "What Is Nattokinase?" *VeryWell,* January 6, 2015. www
.verywell.com/what-is-nattokinase-89831 (accessed April 25, 2017).

Worldhealth.net. "Positive Lifestyle Changes May Lengthen Telomeres."
October 14, 2013. www.worldhealth.net/news/positive-lifestyle-changes
-may-lengthen-telomeres/ (accessed May 2, 2017).

Worldhealth.net. "Shrinking Telomeres May Foretell Dementia." August 24,
2012. www.worldhealth.net/news/shrinking-telomeres-may-foretell-dementia
(accessed April 25, 2017).

Worldhealth.net. "Telomere Restoration Reverses Aging-Related Disease."
December 7, 2010. www.worldhealth.net/news/telomere-restoration-reverses
-aging-related-diseas/ (accessed April 25, 2017).

Veracity, Dani. "Essential Fatty Acid Phosphatidylserine (PS) Is Powerful
Prevention for Memory Loss, Alzheimer's and Dementia." *Natural News,*
January 9, 2006. www.naturalnews.com/016646_Phosphatidylserine
_Alzheimers.html (accessed April 25, 2017).

10

ADAPTOGENS

The What, the Why, the How

"Healing," papa would tell me, "is not a science, but the intuitive art of wooing nature."

W. H. AUDEN

No matter what she did, Susan found that she always felt a little depressed and experienced feelings of stress. She had been to many doctors, almost all of whom had prescribed antidepressants and counseling. Even though she followed this advice, nothing seemed to work for her. Susan always felt stressed, and down and out.

One day, she came across an article about adaptogens and how they can be used to help treat stress and depression. With all other forms of treatment exhausted, Susan had nothing to lose. She went to a natural grocer and found a few that were recommended in the article. In just a few weeks, Susan felt her entire mood turn around!

Have you found that when you go to the doctor they always prescribe something to ease the symptoms rather than cure the underlying cause? Depression is one of the most diagnosed mental illnesses. If you were to ask many of the people you are around on a daily basis, you would find that many are suffering from depression symptoms. While antidepressant medication can help ease the symptoms, it is often only a temporary fix.

While there are many different forms of depression and just as many causes, it is crucial to note that not all depression can be treated with medication and counseling. Sometimes, there is something off in your body that needs to get back to its natural state of being. As Susan found out, adaptogens have been said to provide relief from depression symptoms. How does this happen? How can you find such relief for yourself?

In this chapter, I am going to give you an introduction to adaptogens and how they can be beneficial as a natural remedy for depression symptoms. I will look at the uses, the benefits, and how each individual adaptogen can be used to ease your stress and depression.

WHAT IS AN ADAPTOGEN?

Since ancient times, adaptogens have helped increase people's health and well-being by helping treat stress and depression and offering other wonderful benefits. Adaptogens occur naturally, and they are easy to implement into one's diet. Those who take them feel better and age better.

Adaptogens help your body and mind to balance themselves.

Before I go into how these substances can have an impact on your life, we need to understand what they are and how they work. By definition, adaptogens are compounds or herbs that are used to help your body maintain homeostasis and thus react better to adverse circumstances. They are often said to do this by acting in a nonspecific way on body systems. There are a variety of natural adaptogens that have shown their healing benefits.

An adaptogen is said to react with the parts of your brain that control how you process stress and feelings of depression. By taking these on a regular basis, you can help prevent stress and depression and live a calmer and more fulfilling lifestyle.

HOW CAN THEY AFFECT YOU?

Adaptogens are said to react with the neurotransmitters of the brain, helping you to psychologically reach a natural balance of emotions. These substances are natural and a great way to help you feel better without conventional medications.

If you are feeling stressed, depressed, or even just emotionally off, adaptogens can help you regain a stable mental and physical state. As mentioned in the last chapter, telomere shortening can occur due to stress and that can lead to premature aging of the body. The good news is that telomere shortening can be reversed. Our bodies are in a constant state of renewal and by adopting a healthy lifestyle you can go from an unhealthy body to a healthy body in as little as a year! And adaptogens can help you in this by helping you deal with stress and depression.

Let's take a look at some of the most popular adaptogens that can help you find balance in your life and how they can have an effect on your wellness.

RHODIOLA ROSEA

The first adaptogen that I feel is worth discussion is *Rhodiola rosea*. This substance is also known as arctic root or golden root. It grows at high altitude in the cold regions of the northern hemisphere in Russia, China, the United States, and Canada.

Uses
In Russian and Scandinavian medicine, it has traditionally been used to increase physical endurance, fight fatigue and depression, and for a handful of other purposes. This herb has been touted as a great way to treat major depression and is becoming more commonly used in treating the illness. In Siberia and Eastern China, the herb has been used for decades in treating depression.

Benefits
There are numerous benefits to taking *Rhodiola rosea,* including:

- Ability to feel it working almost immediately
- Decreases fatigue
- Lessens general anxiety
- Increases mental performance

- Relieves pain
- Treats cancer
- Prohibits stress hormones, making feelings of extreme stress less likely
- Can extend longevity by years
- Protects muscles during physical exercise
- Regulates blood sugars

When taken regularly, it has proven to be just as effective as clinical antidepressants, if not more so.

ASTRAGALUS ROOT (TA-65)

Just like the other adaptogens, astragalus root helps in the regeneration of telomeres and the increase in the feelings of vitality. It too has been found in areas in Asia and has been used for centuries by the population there. Alternative medicine is beginning to discover its benefits, and it is becoming increasingly popular in the United States.

Uses
Astragalus root is an herb that has been used in the strengthening of immunity and physical resistance. If your immune system is weakened or compromised, the use of astragalus root may help prevent you from getting ill as frequently.

Benefits
Astragalus root has its list of benefits. Those taking astragalus root have reported the following:

- Becoming ill less often
- Finding it easier to recover from illnesses
- Having increased eyesight
- Having more energy on a daily basis
- Seeing better control in blood sugars

The supplement has also been shown to improve the lengthening of telomeres, assisting in rebuilding the protective caps and aiding in the reversal of the aging process.

ASHWAGANDHA (INDIAN GINSENG)

Ashwagandha's technical name is *Withania somnifera*. It is also known by the name of poison gooseberry or winter cherry. It is the root of the plant that is used in herbal medicine and is known as Indian ginseng.

Uses

Ashwagandha is used to treat anxiety, increase energy, stamina, and endurance, strengthen the immune system, and promote longevity. Like other adaptogens, it is popular in Asia and has been used for centuries to help with many common conditions that one may experience on a day-to-day basis.

Benefits

Since ashwagandha has been used for centuries, there have been thousands, if not millions of testimonies to its benefits. These benefits include, but are not limited to:

- Treating a wide array of physical ailments
- Reducing stress
- Rejuvenation
- Increased strength and vigor
- Can be grown worldwide
- Enhances athletic performance

Having many of these benefits right at our fingertips can assist us in deciding whether or not taking this supplement is right for us. Its benefits seem great within themselves, so if you're looking for more energy and a natural way to treat your stress, then this might be for you.

BENEFITS OF TAKING AN ADAPTOGEN

Adaptogens work with the body. Sensing when stress levels or other levels are out of whack, they rush to the rescue and return these to normal levels. They don't have any major side effects and are fairly harmless. So you can take more than one adaptogen at a time. Taking whatever serves your personal health needs can decrease the need for clinical pharmaceuticals.

FINDING AN ADAPTOGEN THAT WORKS FOR YOU

Because every person is different, each and every individual has his or her own dietary and psychological needs in order to feel well. With that said, when determining what adaptogens would be right for you, take a look at your health and see what you can benefit from. If you suffer from stress and depression, you may want to use a supplement that will help ease those symptoms.

Adaptogens are also safe to take in combination with one another. If you know that one will offer some of what you need and another will complete the process, it is safe to take more than one at the same time. People who have taken adaptogens for years have found that combining several has yielded more desirable health benefits. Like any other supplement, it is a good idea to consult a health care professional before taking an adaptogen.

POINTS TO REMEMBER

As we take a look at ways to increase our health and vitality, we have come across the supplements of adaptogens. These herbs and substances have great health benefits and date back to ancient times. Many people find that they suffer from stress and depression frequently. It comes from living in a culture where everything needs to be done yesterday. However, we don't need to feel the adverse health effects associated with these conditions.

These supplements have been proven to stop the deterioration of telomeres, the caps that protect chromosomes, and have actually helped in restoring them. This helps slow down the aging process.

Taking adaptogens can be done safely as a supplement and can provide relief from stress, depression, and even help treat chronic illnesses in a natural and safe way. Taking the time to find an adaptogen that will help your individual health needs can increase your longevity and vitality. Knowing that they are time proven, you can feel safe taking them to help boost your mood and ease your stress levels.

We all want to feel less stressed and have more energy, right? Adaptogens can offer these feelings in a natural way!

REFERENCES FOR CHAPTER 10

Alban, Deane. "Stress, Telomeres, and the Secret to Prevent Aging." *Wake Up World,* May 11, 2014. http://wakeup-world.com/2014/05/12/stress-telomeres-and-the-secret-to-prevent-aging/ (accessed May 2, 2017).

Bechtel, Jonathan. "Astragalus: It Stops Aging, Cancer, and More!" Health Kismet Blog, July 13, 2012. http://blog.healthkismet.com/astragalus-health-benefits (accessed May 2, 2017).

ClickOrlando.com. "Secret Formula May Be Key to Reverse Aging," *News6 Orlando,* July 04, 2012. www.clickorlando.com/health/secret-formula-may-be-key-to-reverse-aging (accessed May 2, 2017).

Doss, Angela. "Five Ways Astragalus Helps Your Body Heal Itself." *Natural News,* December 7, 2012. www.naturalnews.com/038251_astragalus_healing_Eastern_medicine.html (accessed May 2, 2017).

The Dr. Oz Show. "Astragalus Root: Is This Right for You?" October 25, 2012. www.doctoroz.com/article/astragalus-root-right-you (accessed May 2, 2017).

Fox, Romy. "Psychodermatology." *LifeExtension,* July 2009. www.lifeextension.com/Magazine/2009/7/Psychodermatology/Page-01 (accessed May 2, 2017).

Health Freedom Alliance. "7 Things You Didn't Know About . . . Ashwagandha!" July 8, 2014. www.healthfreedoms.org/7-things-you-didnt-know-aboutashwagandha/ (accessed May 2, 2017).

Health Freedom Alliance. "How Your Body Rebuilds Itself in Less Than 365 Days!" January 6, 2016. www.healthfreedoms.org/how-your-body-rebuilds-itself-in-less-than-365-days/ (accessed May 2, 2017).

HerbWisdom.com. "Rhodiola Benefits & Information (RhodiolaRosea)." www.herbwisdom.com/herb-rhodiola.html (accessed May 2, 2017).

Jockers, David. "The Immune Boosting Power of Astragalus." *Natural News,* September 27, 2013. www.naturalnews.com/042240_astragalus_immune_boosting_power_adaptogenic_herbs.html (accessed May 2, 2017).

Jones, Derrell. "Help Reverse Aging with Telomere Support." *Natural News,* September 29, 2012. www.naturalnews.com/037360_aging_telomere_longevity.html (accessed May 2, 2017).

Kilham, Chris. "Rhodiolarosea: Nature's Antidepressant." *Fox News Health,* September 10, 2012. www.foxnews.com/health/2012/03/07/rhodiola-rosea-natures-anti-depressant.html (accessed May 2, 2017).

Lipman, Frank. "Adaptogens: Nature's Miracle Anti-stress and Fatigue Fighters."

Be Well Blog, November 13, 2012. www.drfranklipman.com/adaptogens
-natures-miracle-anti-stress-and-fatigue-fighters/ (accessed May 2, 2017).

Mercola, Joseph. "'Golden Root' Adaptogen Used by Russian Cosmonauts and
Athletes and Even the Vikings?" *Mercola,* October 4, 2013. http://products
.mercola.com/rhodiola-extract/ (accessed May 2, 2017).

Perelman School of Medicine at the University of Pennsylvania. "Roseroot Herb
Shows Promise as Potential Depression Treatment Option." *Science Daily,*
March 26, 2015. www.sciencedaily.com/releases/2015/03/150326112336
.htm (accessed May 2, 2017).

Scutti, Susan. "How Long Will I Live? Your Lifespan Depends on Cellular Death
and Progress of Future Science." *Medical Daily,* December 22, 2015. www
.medicaldaily.com/pulse/how-long-will-i-live-your-lifespan-depends-cellular
-death-and-progress-future-science-366480 (accessed May 2, 2017).

Woods, Susan. "TA-65 Featured in Suzanne Somers' New Book, *Bombshell:
Explosive Medical Secrets That Will Redefine Aging.*" *Business Wire,* May 9,
2012. www.businesswire.com/news/home/20120509005471/en/TA-65
-Featured-Suzanne-Somers'-Book-Bombshell-Explosive (accessed May 2,
2017).

Wright, Carolanne. "Leap Tall Buildings in a Single Bound with Rhodiola Herb."
Natural News, September 28, 2012. www.naturalnews.com/037345_rhodiola
_vitality_endurance.html (accessed May 2, 2017).

11

HORMONES
Maintaining Your Inner Balance

I balance my hormones with bioidentical hormones.

SUZANNE SOMERS

I've seen estrogen make princesses out of witches.

MARIA HOAG, MBA

Hormones fill us with the music of life. With proper levels of hormones, there is no end to how good life can feel and what we can accomplish. When hormones are abundant and balanced, we feel young.

When Bernice came for her first appointment, she was in her seventies. She said, "I feel so old!" If truth be told, she looked a lot older than her years. She was extremely wrinkled and lethargic. I spoke to her about hormones, but she was concerned about taking them because her sister had died of breast cancer.

I informed her that all hormones were not alike and sent her to a physician who specialized in bio-identical hormone replacement therapy. When she came for her follow-up appointment she said, "I feel so much better on hormone replacement therapy. It feels like I have been given a new lease on life, and best of all, my sex drive came back!"

As you age, you will notice that no matter how much organic food you eat, how many supplements you take, or how much exercise you get, vibrant health will elude you unless your hormones are at optimal levels and balanced.

> **One of the hallmarks of aging is a decline in hormone levels.**

I am sure you have noticed that some people age faster than others and that two people who are the same age can look much younger or older than their contemporaries. You probably have just attributed this to genetics, but the source can be much greater than that. Hormones have a lot to do with how we age.

One of the hallmarks of aging is a decline in hormone levels. Production of estrogen, progesterone, testosterone, thyroid, DHEA, melatonin, human growth hormone, and other hormones taper off after people reach their twenties and thirties, and many experts agree that age-related hormone deficiencies contribute to the signs and symptoms of aging.

If you have noticed that you just haven't felt right lately, it could be due to the imbalance of your hormones. This might sound scary, but it is actually treatable. Many physicians now specialize in bio-identical hormone replacement therapy. The premise behind this is that by restoring hormone levels to what they were in one's prime, health and vitality improve.

In this chapter, we will examine the main hormones of aging, how they can affect your health, and what you can do about them.

HORMONES AND YOU

In some respects, we think of hormones as something that affects us during puberty and old age. However, hormones are ever present in our daily lives. While we cannot see their immediate effects, when they are imbalanced, we can feel some severe health consequences. In this section, I would like to give you a better idea of what exactly hormones do and how you can recognize them in your own body.

What Do Hormones Do?

Hormones are bodily chemicals that regulate our moods, body cycles, and stimulate our cells into performing as they are meant to. If your hormones are not in balance, you can feel fatigued and just not well. Learning which hormones are important to your gender and age group and how they affect you can really help you to identify a hormonal imbalance.

When Hormones Begin to Change

At certain stages in our lives, it is inevitable that we will deal with hormonal changes. We see this all the time with children entering puberty or women entering menopause. The hormones are changing. While they increase or decrease, the body may go through subtle or extreme changes. Teenagers experience mood changes while menopausal women might experience hot flashes. These are just a few of the side effects of hormones changing as we age.

Hormones can also change for other reasons that are directly linked to your lifestyle and health. Not all people recognize these changes, but they can have a dynamic effect on your daily life if left untreated. Recognizing hormonal changes will help you and your doctors find the best treatment options so that you can feel well and age well.

Hormonal Changes and Your Overall Health

From your thyroid to your growth hormones, there is a constant flow of hormones moving through your body. While I am only focusing on the hormones that deal with aging, any hormonal imbalance can drastically affect your overall health. Due to the fact that hormones are often overlooked, you may be suffering from an imbalance and not even know that it is the reason why you don't feel well.

While we expect hormones to change at certain periods of our lives, it is possible for them to change at any time. These changes can affect your mood, physical wellness, and quality of life. This makes it important to identify hormonal imbalances before they become a more serious problem.

Freda was referred to me by her internist. She had just gone through menopause without it being a problem. She ate really well, often having vegetables even for breakfast, and took a lot of supplements. She said, "I feel something is missing, I just can't explain it, but it's as if my high energy level and love of life have been diminished."

I went through a check list of questions I have for my patients and ascertained that she was lacking in estrogen because she was experiencing vaginal dryness. I sent her to a physician who could test her hormones and she was prescribed transdermal estrogen. When she came back she told me with a smile on her face that she now has a new boyfriend.

Signs of Hormonal Imbalance

I have touched upon a few of the symptoms of imbalanced hormones. The symptoms are different for many people, and a hormonal imbalance can sometimes go unidentified for years. Knowing your body and helping yourself by finding these signs will help you to get treatment faster and return to your former standard of health.

> **Mood swings could be a sign of hormonal imbalance.**

Signs of hormonal imbalances include mood changes, fatigue, changes in appetite, sleep disturbances, memory loss, changes in eating habits, headaches, and a multitude of other annoyances. If you have found that you are acting or feeling differently, you may have a hormonal imbalance to blame.

WHAT ARE THE MAIN HORMONES RESPONSIBLE FOR AGING?

As I mentioned before, there are hormones throughout your body that control many different functions. What I hope to give you in this chapter are the main hormones that play a role in aging and how they can affect your health. Since this book focuses on longevity and healthy aging, it would be an extreme disservice to leave out hormones and their effects on aging.

Estrogen

Estrogen is essentially how three main types of hormones are referred to in the female body. Estradiol, estrone, and estriol, all comprise what we know of as the hormone estrogen. The production of this hormone is important in women because it supplies the feminine traits. It is suppressed until puberty, when a young girl will start to see its effects on her mind and body.

Estrogen is very important for the female body.

How It Affects You

Estrogen is very important in the formation of the female body. It affects all of the major organs as well as aiding in reproduction. There are dire consequences of having too much or not enough of this hormone in the body. Older women often have to take hormone replacements to make sure their body has enough estrogen to keep it from developing diseases such as osteoporosis.

You may have heard how the lack of estrogen can affect an older woman, but estrogen deficiency is also common at a younger age. In the late twenties and later, if a woman experiences a deficiency of this hormone, she can be plagued with migraine headaches and other symptoms.

When to Seek Help

Having a deficiency of estrogen can cause some major health problems in women. One of the signs of being deficient in estrogen is memory loss. Those who suffer from Alzheimer's and dementia often have a lack of estrogen. If you suddenly notice that you are having trouble remembering or that you commonly drop your thoughts, then it may be a sign that you might want to get your estrogen levels checked.

Estrogen Dominance

Estrogen dominance occurs when the body produces more estrogen than it does progesterone. This puts the body off balance. One may experience bleeding, cramps, weight gain, and intestinal discomfort. This condition can be battled by taking a progesterone supplement or cream.

Many women are misled into thinking that estrogen can cause cancer and therefore refuse to take it to ease menopausal discomfort, but it is important to know that of the three estrogens, estriol is the safest and can be compounded into a cream or pill by a compounding pharmacy. In fact, Japanese women who have the lowest incidence of breast cancer in the world are quite high in estriol. Sadly enough, estriol is often overlooked in favor of the other two forms of estrogen. In fact, estriol can actually help to prevent breast cancer!

Progesterone

While this hormone is commonly associated with pregnancy, it is responsible for a large share of one's well-being. Progesterone is produced by the ovaries. Larger amounts are produced when pregnancy occurs in order to protect the developing fetus. However, progesterone is important for much more than a healthy pregnancy.

The hormones progesterone and estrogen complement each other and serve to help the body stay balanced. When the body lacks these hormones, a substitute hormone, cortisol, is produced, which has proven to be harmful if produced in excess. Let's look at the ways the hormone progesterone is extremely important to health.

Why It's Important

Aside from protecting a forming fetus, progesterone plays a large role in stress relief and aging. As mentioned, if the body doesn't produce enough of this hormone, it begins to produce cortisol, which can be potentially harmful, even though it serves a purpose similar to progesterone. In fact, a decrease in progesterone is believed to be responsible for osteoporosis. Those who are being treated for a progesterone deficiency sometimes see a reversal in their osteoporosis symptoms.

The benefits of progesterone include:

- Relief from anxiety
- Improved memory
- Protection of brain cells
- Preventing seizures
- Aiding in respiration
- Helping to prevent and treat cancers

With so many benefits, it is important to know when your body is lacking this hormone so that you can get help replacing it in your body. Not only does it help with certain conditions, but it can also aid in the aging process. If the skin becomes dry and wrinkled, you are more than likely lacking progesterone and need to find a replacement for it.

Pregnenolone

This hormone is found in both genders, mainly during the puberty years. Like progesterone in women, it helps regulate stress and balance out the hormones of the body. While it is still relatively new in the research of hormones, pregnenolone is found to be a very beneficial hormone for regulating other hormones. Pregnenolone can be purchased over the counter.

What Does It Do?

While progesterone is helpful in larger amounts, the hormones of estrogen and cortisol can be harmful in large amounts. Pregnenolone is responsible for helping regulate the balance of these possibly caustic hormones.

Not only does it protect the body from excess hormonal damage, but it is also a hormone that helps the brain. It is said to aid in increasing memory and reducing stress in middle-aged and older adults. As for aging, this hormone acts as a natural "facelift." Pregnenolone helps aid blood flow to the skin, helping the skin retain its elasticity.

Testosterone

Testosterone is a hormone that is linked to personality and sex drive. It helps with assertiveness, motivation, and a feeling of control. While both men and women produce this hormone, it is produced in greater amounts in men. In women, it is part of battling the aging process, and increases after menopause.

If a woman lacks testosterone, she may feel fatigued, unmotivated, and experience health problems. A deficiency of testosterone is linked to memory loss, Alzheimer's, osteoporosis, heart attacks, and other severe symptoms. A woman with too much testosterone will start to show manly characteristics, such as facial hair.

DHEA

DHEA is one of the most important regulatory hormones in your body. Taking a look at DHEA and all of its functions will help you to appreciate it more and allow you to recognize the importance of keeping it in balance.

What Does It Do?

Produced in the adrenal gland, DHEA is responsible for the regulation of at least eighteen steroid hormones in your body. That's a huge responsibility! You find this hormone mainly in your blood stream and skin. The production of this hormone is at its highest in our midtwenties and dips when we are reaching the age of seventy.

> **Lack of DHEA causes dry and wrinkled skin in the elderly.**

DHEA can be transitioned into whatever hormone your body needs at the time. So, if you're experiencing a shortage of hormones such as estrogen, testosterone, or progesterone, DHEA can come to the rescue and become these hormones. This makes DHEA a pro-hormone and an incredibly important one to maintaining hormonal balance within the body.

The absence of DHEA is responsible for the dry and wrinkled skin that is commonly associated with elderly adults. This can be a sign also that you are experiencing an imbalance of the hormone. Let's take a look at this important hormone and how it can affect overall well-being.

Health Problems Associated with DHEA Deficiency

When the body is low on DHEA, you may be at risk for coronary heart disease. In fact, this is one of the signs of the disease. Since DHEA is very important to health, it is important that you understand the benefits of having a sufficient amount of DHEA in your body.

DHEA has many benefits including:

- Reduces the risk of cardiovascular disease
- Lowers the levels of cortisol in the body

- Helps repair damaged systems
- Prevents bone deterioration
- Increases immunity
- Decreases risk of stroke

Those who lack DHEA tend to look and feel frail. When noticing weakness or other symptoms of a hormonal imbalance, get to your doctor right away. It can make a huge difference in your overall health and well-being.

How to Notice an Imbalance

As with any hormonal imbalance, you will notice some signs that your DHEA is off. This may be feeling tired, having dull and brittle skin, or having digestive problems. While there might be many causes for these symptoms, it is a good sign that maybe your body is experiencing a hormonal imbalance. Talk to your doctor if you feel like you may be experiencing any sort of hormone imbalance.

Is an Imbalance Safe to Treat?

DHEA can be taken every day. It can be found over the counter in an oral supplement or a cream that can be applied to the skin. This can help to significantly reduce the skin symptoms that a lack of the hormone can cause. Many people apply this hormone topically on a daily basis! Doctors have been able to give large amounts of this hormone without any adverse effects. However, it is good to be cautious taking it if you are pregnant or breastfeeding, and one should get a blood test to ascertain the amount of DHEA that is needed.

Oxytocin

Oxytocin is often referred to as the "love" hormone. It is secreted whenever we feel love or attraction to another being. It is also secreted when a woman is breastfeeding. It is important to know about this hormone, as it is a powerful antidepressant. It is also linked to blood pressure and sex drive.

How Does It Affect Your Health?

A lack of oxytocin can have severe effects upon your intimacy and love life. It also has a huge role in pregnancy and child delivery. This may be the reason that a new mother can forget the immense pain of childbirth.

Studies have shown that oxytocin is linked to helping in pain relief; this is very helpful to older adults who experience chronic pain. It is also said to reduce stress and help aid in sexual relationships.

KNOWING IF YOU ARE EXPERIENCING A HORMONE IMBALANCE

Hormone loss is a normal part of life. Look at women who are experiencing menopause. The amounts of estrogen and progesterone drastically decrease during this period of time, often making it necessary to use hormone replacement therapy.

> **Old age isn't the only time you can experience hormone imbalance.**

Older age isn't the only time that you may notice your hormones changing. Young women experience cycles of hormone production on a monthly basis associated with their menstrual cycle. How can you tell that your hormones are out of whack? Generally, symptoms of hormone imbalance include:

- Fatigue
- Mood changes
- Trouble sleeping
- Changes in weight and appetite
- Frailty

These are not all of the symptoms, but they are the most common ones that are experienced. Also, look for skin changes, as a lack of certain hormones can affect the appearance of your skin.

TREATING HORMONE IMBALANCES: NATURE VERSUS MODERN MEDICINE

In the past, hormone imbalances were difficult to identify and treat. However, with advances in modern medicine, hormone imbalances are easier to treat, making it easier for those who experience them to obtain supplements.

Having a good balance of hormones is important in the aging process. As I have mentioned several times in this chapter, a lack of certain hormones can have a huge effect on the skin, making it look older than it really needs to. Hormonal skin creams can allow you to look and feel better as you age. They will help to replenish hormones that are being lost during the aging process.

Allowing nature to have its way could lead to an early death. It doesn't have to be this way. With modern medical advances, it is now possible to supplement the hormones you lack in order to balance out your system. This can lead to slowing down the aging process and allowing your skin and bones to remain strong and vital as you age chronologically.

POINTS TO REMEMBER

Hormones can affect your overall health. Not only do they affect your mood, but they can affect the way in which you age and how you look as you age.

The main hormones that are associated with aging, estrogen, progesterone, pregnenolone, testosterone, DHEA, and oxytocin, have all proven to aid in youthful appearances when taken as a supplement.

When hormones are out of balance, you can experience many symptoms, from mental to physical disturbances. Taking supplements can help you feel and look better and increase your chances at a longer and more fulfilling life.

Hormones are extremely important in a person's overall health. They affect the body's main systems, regulate mood, and prevent serious diseases. We may not notice the immediate symptoms of a hormonal imbalance, but once it is identified, there are wonderful advances in modern medicine that can help regulate hormone levels.

Knowing and understanding the youth hormones can aid you in finding solutions to common health problems and seeking help in making sure that you are in balance. I encourage you to get your hormone levels checked and be watchful for symptoms of a hormonal imbalance.

REFERENCES FOR CHAPTER 11

Cole, William. "7 Hormone Imbalances That Could Explain Your Fatigue, Moodiness & Weight Gain." *MindBodyGreen,* February 10, 2016. www .mindbodygreen.com/0-23636/7-hormone-imbalances-that-could-explain -your-fatigue-moodiness-weight-gain.html (accessed May 4, 2017).

Dotinga, Randy. "Hormones Might Offer Relief from Chronic Pain, Small Study Suggests." *HealthDay,* March 8, 2014. http://consumer.healthday .com/women-s-health-information-34/misc-hormones-health-news-390 /hormones-might-offer-relief-from-chronic-pain-small-study-suggests-685576 .html (accessed May 4, 2017).

Empower Pharmacy. "Oxytocin Nasal Spray." https://empower.pharmacy/drugs /oxytocin-nasal-spray.html (accessed May 4, 2017).

Endocrine Society. "Cortisol: Stress Hormone Linked to Frailty." *Science Daily,* February 20, 2014. www.sciencedaily.com/releases/2014/02/140220131349 .htm (accessed May 4, 2017).

Gabriel, E. "DHEA: The Mother Hormone." *Green Willow Tree.* www .greenwillowtree.com/dhea/?___store=default (accessed May 4, 2017).

Health Freedom Alliance. "9 Signs of Hormone Imbalance That Most Women Mistakenly Ignored." www.healthfreedoms.org/9-signs-of-hormone -imbalance-that-most-women-mistakenly-ignored/ (accessed May 4, 2017).

HealthySkin Solutions. "DHEA." November 18, 2015. www.healthyskinsolutions .com/dhea/ (accessed May 4, 2017).

Lee, John R. "Estrogen Dominance: An Elevated Estradiol to Progesterone Ratio." John R. Lee, M.D., July 12, 2014. www.johnleemd.com/estrogen -dominance.html (accessed May 4, 2017).

Mercola, Joseph. "The Links Between Your Diet and Hormone Levels." *Mercola,* February 23, 2014. http://articles.mercola.com/sites/articles /archive/2014/02/23/hormones.aspx (accessed May 4, 2017).

———. "Keep Aging Parents Happy, Healthy and Independent with Bioidentical

Hormones." *Natural News,* March 23, 2009. www.naturalnews.com/025915 _hormones_aging_WHO.html (accessed May 4, 2017).

Natural Medicines Comprehensive Database. "DHEA: MedlinePlus Supplements." *MedlinePlus,* August 15, 2014. www.nlm.nih.gov/medlineplus /druginfo/natural/331.html (accessed May 4, 2017).

Peat, Raymond. "Progesterone Pregnenolone and DHEA: Three Youth-Associated Hormones." RayPeat, July 28, 2013. http://raypeat.com/articles/articles /three-hormones.shtml (accessed May 4, 2017).

Post, Bryan. "How Does Oxytocin Lessen the Stress and Bring on the Sex?" *Oxcytocin Central,* July 5, 2011. http://oxytocincentral.com/2011/07/how-does -oxytocin-lessen-the-stress-and-bring-on-the-sex/ (accessed May 4, 2017).

SmartPublications. "Oxytocin: The Real Love Hormone!" www.smart-publications .com/articles/oxytocin-the-real-love-hormone/ (accessed May 4, 2017).

Smith, Timothy J. "DHEA." From *Renewal: The Anti-aging Revolution* (New York: Rodale Press, 1998). Website of Clif Arrington, M.D., August 17, 2014. www.anti-agingmd.com/dhea.html (accessed May 4, 2017).

Stokel, Kirk. "New Research Substantiates the Anti-aging Properties of DHEA." *LifeExtension,* December, 2010. www.lifeextension.com/Magazine/2010/12 /New-Research-Substantiates-the-Anti-Aging-Properties-of-DHEA/Page-01 (accessed May 4, 2017).

UT Southwestern Medical Center. "Scientists Find Estrogen Promotes Blood-Forming Stem Cell Function." *Science Daily,* January 22, 2014. www.sciencedaily .com/releases/2014/01/140122133419.htm (accessed May 4, 2017).

Whitaker, Julian. "Natural Bioidentical Hormones." Whitaker Wellness Institute Medical Clinic, October, 2015. www.whitakerwellness.com/therapies /natural-bioidentical-hormones/ (accessed May 4, 2017).

WorldHealth.net. "Low DHEA Predicts Coronary Heart Disease." December 8, 2015. www.worldhealth.net/news/low-dhea-predicts-coronary-heart-disease (accessed May 4, 2017).

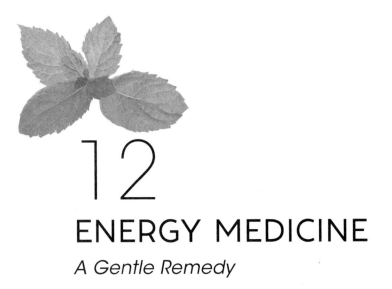

12

ENERGY MEDICINE
A Gentle Remedy

If you want to find the secret of the universe, think in terms of energy, frequency, and vibration.

NIKOLA TESLA

There is a force in the universe, which if we permit it, will flow through us and produce miraculous results.

GANDHI

As a health care practitioner for the last thirty years in Southern California, I have always been interested in health, not only for myself, but for my patients. My education and practice of homeopathy and flower remedies have led me to understand that we are really energetic beings. My exposure to the benefits of acupuncture and Chinese medicine has taught me about the concept of *qi* or *chi*—energy circulating through our bodies. For this reason, I have not only used energy medicine in my practice, but in my personal life. These are some of the changes that I have observed:

- Increased energy
- Improved immunity
- Quicker recovery from injury
- Amelioration of pain
- More organized thinking
- Immediate solution to problems
- Life seems to flow more effortlessly
- A relaxed sense of "allowing"
- Being in the right place at the right time
- Much more synchronicity

> **I believe that energy medicine is one of the best things you can do for anti-aging.**

I believe that energy medicine is one of the best things one can do as one ages to help regenerate the body by eliminating energy blockages, both mentally and physically, thereby allowing the free flow of qi, which I have come to believe is the real secret behind vitality and vibrant health.

Did you ever wonder why some people look and feel a lot older than their years and why it is that some people are burdened with chronic illness as they age, while others aren't? Why is it that some people continue to remain young, energetic, happy, vital, and productive as they get older? Could there be factors other than diet, exercise, and supplementation that contribute to the quality of life as one ages?

I have found that there is a lot more to keeping the body and mind healthy than what we take in, in terms of food and supplements. When I began my practice thirty years ago, I worked in an office that exposed me to the concept that we are really energetic beings and if that energy is permitted to flow without obstruction, the body has an amazing ability to heal itself. I was exposed to acupuncture, and later homeopathy, and witnessed and experienced the power that they possessed in healing. In this chapter, we will be discussing three different types of energy medicine and how it can help you to look and feel better, no matter where you are in life.

Energy healing or energy medicine promotes healing by enhancing energy flow and correcting disturbances in the "human energy field" that surrounds the body and flows through it; it supports the self-healing and regenerating capacity of one's own body.

> **The body's ability to heal is greater than they
> have ever permitted you to believe.**

Traditional Chinese medicine, homeopathy, and Bach flower remedies all work on the same principle, which is enhancing energy by addressing the distortion of the vital force. These ancient healing modalities are beginning to gain more attention. Currently, there is a kind of revival of ancient understandings about energy healing in the light of modern science.

Energy medicine operates under the principle that health is determined by the overall flow and balance of a person's vital life force or energy. Imbalances or blockages in the natural flow of this subtle energy field of the body are the true cause of illness. In this chapter, we will examine the ancient and time-proven practices of acupuncture, qigong, homeopathy, and flower remedies. These all help to restore energetic flow. We will also look at how they work and how you can use them to enhance your own chi, qi, prana, or energy to activate your self-healing mechanisms.

HOW ENERGY MEDICINE CAN HEAL

When all your energies are brought into harmony, your body flourishes. And when your body flourishes, your soul has a soil in which it can blossom in the world. These are the ultimate reasons for energy medicine—to prepare the soil and nurture the blossom.

DONNA EDEN,
*ENERGY MEDICINE: BALANCING YOUR BODY'S
ENERGIES FOR OPTIMAL HEALTH, JOY, AND VITALITY*

The goal of energy medicine is to channel your energy in order to strengthen, regenerate, and heal your body. If you have tried just about everything, I encourage you to read this chapter with an open mind and see if this might be a solution to your problems.

What Is Energy Medicine?

> *Your illness is NOT your fault, but your healing IS your responsibility.*
>
> Donna Eden

Before you can use energy medicine efficiently, you need to understand what it is. The simplest way to describe energy medicine is to understand that your body is full of natural energy. In Eastern medicine, these are referred to in various ways, including auras, chakras, chi, qi, or prana. These are just different names for the same vital energy or life force that flows through the body. Don't let the different names confuse you. They have different names because they were developed in different cultures and there was no standardization back then like there is today. What's important is that in all these ancient energy medicine systems, it is said that this energy needs to flow freely through your body in order for you to feel whole and healthy.

When your energy paths are blocked, that is when you feel unwell as you lack energy. According to energy medicine, it is important to unblock these disturbances in order to feel happier and healthier. In the next section, we are going to take a look at how energy medicine works and how it can help you to feel better. There are many different ways to support energy medicine, and I will also cover these in this chapter. But first, let's take a look at how energy medicine works and how it can help you to regain your stamina and health.

How Does It Work?

In many cultures, there are practices that are used to help unblock the energy channels and return the flow of energy to where it should be. In her article about her energy medicine experience, Wendy Adamson talks about her experience with the practice of Maori healing. She had been suffering immense neurological pain, and all of her medical tests had come back normal. When she visited Shari, a former supermodel turned Maori healer, she finally found the relief that she had been seeking. Her energy channels had been blocked.

Wendy submitted to the Maori healing, a practice of New Zealand. After the process had been completed, she felt peaceful and happy. Ever since then, she has opened up her mind to energy healing. Wendy has been an advocate for what it can do for a person who tries it.

In energy medicine, techniques are used to open up the energy channels that are blocked in your body. This can be done through movement, touch, and aromatherapy. The combination of these methods allows the energy to flow normally through the body once again. As Wendy experienced, it was through the healer's touch that the pain was forced out of her body. While the healer touched her, she encouraged Wendy to give up the pain.

Why Should You Care about Energy Medicine?

Energy medicine is the oldest, safest, most available, most affordable medicine there is.

DONNA EDEN

If you're still not convinced by energy medicine, then you probably want more details about why and how energy medicine can be beneficial to you and your health. After all, energy medicine sounds like some ancient hocus pocus, right? Energy medicine isn't just a hype, however. Even if you cannot attest to its healing qualities, you can still see significant benefits from the practice, such as:

- Changing your outlook on disease and medicine
- Releasing your negative thoughts, memories, and emotions
- Preventing future occurrences of disease
- Enabling your body's healing mechanisms to function properly
- Helping you to connect with nature

These benefits can help you to feel less stressed-out and better able to cope with daily challenges. If you want to prevent getting ill and feel more at ease, what have you got to lose?

Healing Ourselves through Energy

Meredith was recently diagnosed with cancer. She had already had surgery to remove the tumor and was being treated by an orthomolecular physician who gave her hundreds of vitamins as well as frequent vitamin C infusions. She was meditating, doing positive affirmations, along with other relaxation and positivity techniques. Despite all of this, the cancer had metastasized. Meredith felt something was missing.

I explained to her that all illness or "dis-ease" is caused by a distortion of the vital force. There was something that was not letting her heal. It could be environmental, physical, psychological, or spiritual. When she told me her story it became quite clear to me that the "thing" that was holding her back from healing was her low self-esteem.

She was surrounded by highly educated and successful people, and she felt inferior to them because she lacked a college degree. Due to this, she created a false persona, or mask, that she used to convince people that she was just as good as them, maybe even better, but deep down all of her relationships were tainted by the delusion of inferiority and the need to constantly prove her worth. Homeopathy has a perfect remedy for this and she was given it. She recently had a cat scan and there was no trace of cancer in her body.

We all want to be healthy as we grow older. However, in the face of modern technology and medicine, it is more common for people to lose touch with their energy, to relegate their health to an outside person. A connection of your mind, body, and spirit is essential to feeling whole, alive, and healthy. Finding that connection is crucial for your overall health and aging. Where do you find this connection? Let's look at ways in which you can find your mind, body, and spirit connection.

How to Connect Your Mind, Body, and Spirit

First of all, you have to recognize that the world around you is all energy. Everything, from the chair you sit in to the food you eat is just shaped energy. Knowing this, you will be able to see yourself as a combination of many different forms of energy.

Your mind communicates with your body and spirit through your energy channels. If these are blocked or damaged, then your mind, body, and spirit cannot effectively communicate. It is important that these all be able to communicate in order to realize the full potential of your energy. Your mind holds a lot of power over your being. Consciously and subconsciously, you may find that you are unintentionally blocking your connection because of your mind. Learn to free your mind in order to help make this connection more solid.

> **The world around you is all energy.**

Allow your mind, body, and spirit to communicate freely. If one of them is not allowing energy to flow properly, find ways to make this energy flow. It can be the difference in your overall health!

Roberta was sent to me because she had trouble carrying a pregnancy to full term and had miscarriage after miscarriage. Although she already had two children whom she loved dearly, she felt another one wanted to be born. She became pregnant about six months ago, but again lost the child. She felt she had really bonded with this new life in her and told the doctor she wanted to try again. I immediately recognized that her problem was trapped grief and suggested some flower remedies. She did not keep her next appointment, and I didn't see her again until a year later when I went swimming at a local pool. There she was, smiling at me and holding a beautiful infant daughter, the child she was able to carry to full term.

Healing in the Future

With the advances in medicine, we might think that Western medicine will be the solution to all of our health problems. However, the ancient forms of medicine are coming back and proving themselves to be stronger than any medication that a doctor can prescribe you because they treat the cause, not the symptom.

Focusing on your energy and the flow of energy through your body could be the health care of the future. Knowing your body and its energy will help you to be more in tune with yourself and your natural state of being. Let's now discuss some of these promising energy medicine systems that will be part of the healing paradigm in the future.

HOMEOPATHY

Homeopathy is the safest and most reliable approach to ailments and has withstood the assaults of established medical practice for over 100 years.

YEHUDI MENUHIN

As medicine evolves, homeopathy has become more widely recognized. This new medical practice is said to help individuals focus on their own healing abilities rather than relying on modern medicine to do the trick. These healing methods are much different from going to the doctor's office. Let's take a look at what homeopathy is and how it can be the medical care of the future.

When I was working in a clinic in Oxnard several years ago, Paula was referred to me by her physician, who believed that she needed a different approach to her chronic depression, health issues, and lethargy than modern medicine could offer. She was recently diagnosed with type 2 diabetes. Unlike many diabetics, Paula was small, thin, was very physically active, and ate a healthy diet. I couldn't help but wonder what was going on. I began to question her very gently about her family, activities, and when her health problems began. She began to trust me and confide in me, telling me in Spanish that she never got over the death of her only son who was shot outside his house in a gang slaying. This is when everything started.

I immediately saw that her vital energy was depleted through chronic grief. I recommended a high potency constitutional homeopathic remedy that addresses old grief. When she came back for a follow-up visit the next month, she had a smile on her face.

What Is Homeopathy?
With homeopathic medicine, natural substances are used to treat the cause of the problem rather than numbing the symptoms. This can include minerals, herbs, and other natural components that are prepared by dilution and succession to release their energetic power. So there is virtually nothing of the original material substance left, only the molecular imprint. You can find these in either homeopathic pharmacies or even in the over-the-counter medication aisle at your local store. There are many homeopathic remedies on the shelves for common ailments such as the cold and the flu.

In homeopathy, the concept of treatment is treating the person, not the disease. Homeopathic medicine focuses on the origin of the illness, and the cause of it. By taking these factors into consideration, homeopathic practitioners are able to find alternative ways to treat the symptoms. These methods focus on the source of the problem rather than subduing the symptoms.

Those who pursue homeopathic remedies have actually been healed much more effectively and permanently than those who take medications to suppress symptoms.

Do Homeopathic Remedies Work?

Homeopathy cures a greater percentage of cases than any other method of treatment. Homeopathy is the latest and refined method of treating patients economically and nonviolently.

MAHATMA GANDHI

Since we have lived so long in a society that is focused on modern medicine, you may have your doubts about the effectiveness of homeopathic treatments. However, homeopathic medicine is backed by research and scientific evidence. Those who engage in homeopathic medicine report that the condition is cured more often than those who are treated by modern medical procedures. Going to the source of the illness rather than treating its symptoms greatly maximizes the effectiveness of these techniques.

Homeopathic versus Modern Treatments

Since modern health care focuses on symptom suppression, in order to alleviate pain, discomfort, or any other problem, a doctor will, more often than not, prescribe medications that are a combination of man-made components. These often produce debilitating side effects that can be more severe than the original condition.

Homeopathic medicine has no side effects at all!

ACUPUNCTURE

Carla had severe back pain due to a car accident many years ago. She said, "My spine is trashed." She had tried many kinds of injections for the pain through the years and was seriously considering spinal surgery.

Since I worked in an office with a Chinese acupuncturist, I suggested she try that. At first she was very skeptical saying her doctors thought acupuncture was a placebo, I said she had nothing to lose by trying it. It took several sessions, but along with a home yoga practice and acupuncture she became relatively pain free and continues to this day with both, and has avoided surgery.

Acupuncture is an ancient form of treatment that has been practiced in China for over three thousand years. Not only is it becoming much more accepted in the United States in recent years, but physicians are now being trained in medical schools to use it in their practice. As time goes on, practitioners of Western medicine have begun to specialize in the practice of acupuncture. This method has been proven to treat and heal various ailments, from digestive issues to respiratory problems and even emotional problems. Acupuncture is now widely respected and used all over the world from Cuba to Korea, Japan, and South America on people as well as animals.

What Is Acupuncture?

Acupuncture is a medical system based on the theory that there are channels of energy, or meridians, that control the entire body. Imbalance in the energy of these meridians causes all kinds of disease and chronic pain. Acupuncture uses sharp needles that are inserted into the skin at certain specific points to interact with the energy of the meridians and rebalance the system. The difference between acupuncture and allopathic medicine is that it goes after the root cause of the disease while allopathic medicine is mostly focused on symptoms.

> **Acupuncture opens the channels of energy in the body.**

According to the theory of acupuncture there are fourteen major channels or meridians and thousands of smaller channels through which chi energy flows. The acupuncture points act like gates on these channels, and if they are blocked, it can restrict the free flow of chi and result in illness. Acupuncture needles are used to open these gates and allow the energy to flow freely once again. Regular therapy sessions performed for three to four weeks can allow the vital energy to flow and heal the body of whatever illness there might be. The acupuncture points to be activated are chosen based on the illness.

The History of Acupuncture

Acupuncture is thought to have begun in China. The earliest written record of the entire theory of acupuncture is found in *The Yellow Emperor's Classic of Internal Medicine,* which is believed to have been written around 100 BCE. Acupuncture is thought to have been much older than this book and there are signs that other primitive cultures also practiced similar medical techniques as far back as the Bronze Age. A 5,000-year-old mummified body was found near Austria that had fifteen tattoos that corresponded to traditional acupuncture points.

Benefits of Acupuncture

For a long time, acupuncture was considered to simply be superstitious mumbo jumbo or a pseudoscience at best, but there is a growing body of evidence showing that acupuncture does work. A review of all clinical trials on acupuncture was done by the World Health Organization and they found that acupuncture has various effects on the body. Some of these benefits include:

- Stimulation of electromagnetic signals in the body that release immune system cells and pain-killing chemicals
- Stimulation of the hypothalamus and pituitary gland
- Increase in the production of neurotransmitters and neurohormones
- Activation of the body's natural opioid system, which helps in inducing sleep and reducing pain
- Deactivating certain parts of the brain like the limbic system, which is related to processing pain

Based on these studies, now it is believed that acupuncture has the ability to reduce pain. It is used for relief from chronic pain in diseases such as osteoarthritis, headache and migraines, hypertension, low back pain, tennis elbow, neck pain, postoperative pain, and more. It has also been found to work well in patients recovering from radiotherapy and chemotherapy. It helps in reducing nausea and other adverse effects of chemotherapy. It can also be used for depression, stress, recovering from addiction, and any other problem where pain relief is needed.

Acupuncture is a healthier alternative to pain relief drugs because it doesn't cause any side effects and is nonaddictive but also because it is more than just symptom relief. It actually works at the core problem and helps to get rid of pain in the long run. Acupuncture needles are painless when a trained professional is using them. But if you still feel scared of the needles, you can consider acupressure instead.

Acupressure acts on the same principles as acupuncture and targets the same points in the body but instead of using hypodermic needles it uses blunt objects to put pressure on the acupuncture points. Research has shown that even without inserting needles in the body, the pain relief results are similar to acupuncture.

BACH FLOWER REMEDIES

The concept that the mind and emotions can be the cause of illness is not a new one. In fact many physicians have considered the mind to be the major cause of illness. There are many approaches to treating the mind and emotions. One method that people have found beneficial has been Bach flower remedies. These are natural remedies that are in the form of a tincture that is placed under your tongue. They are reputed to balance emotional distress.

How Are Bach Flower Remedies Used?

In his research, Dr. Edward Bach found that combining certain flowers helped to create compounds that would help ease certain emotional states. Dr. Bach found that different combinations of flowers would have different effects. The elements of color and scent also played a huge role in the effectiveness of the tincture. In his transition from Western medicine to homeopathy, he found that flowers had many uses in treating emotional and psychological distress. He tested certain flower essences on those experiencing emotional distress and found that flower essences, when specially prepared, were helpful for dealing with many emotional disturbances that were preventing ease and tranquillity.

With the floral essences, he combined them with brandy to form tinctures to be used for treatment. The tinctures were formed by soaking certain flowers in water or drying them out in sunlight to get their healing components from them. These were then tested on people with certain psychological and emotional issues to find out their effectiveness. The flowers are believed to have energy and vibrations that were significant to the healing process. After much research, Dr. Bach eventually came up with around forty flower remedies that treat guilt, grief, jealousy, being overwhelmed, poor self-image, exhaustion, having no boundaries, and so forth.

I have used and taught doctors to use Bach remedies and even made house calls to cats with behavioral issues.

Do These Tinctures Work?

Although there is no scientific evidence that explains how Bach flower remedies actually work, they do indeed work. They have been used on animals and people all over the world. I have used Bach remedies to treat children and pets with remarkable success. This is not something you need special training to use, but learning about each remedy will lead you to the right one for you.

QIGONG

Energy medicine can address physical illness and emotional or mental disorders, and can also promote high-level wellness and peak performance. It utilizes techniques from healing traditions such as acupuncture, yoga, kinesiology, and qigong. Energy medicine is the science and the art of optimizing your energies to help your body and mind function at their best. Controlling your chemistry by managing your energies is the fast track for helping your body adapt to the challenges of the 21st century.

DONNA EDEN

Qigong is another form of ancient Chinese medicine that has been used for over three thousand years. In fact, most hospitals in China have qigong healing practitioners on their staff.

What Is Qigong?

Qigong is a practice of exercises and movements that improve the energy flow of the body. This method focuses on your movements while concentrating on your body and your breathing. Qigong is said to help you become more in tune with your body's energy and help you to alleviate pain and discomfort.

Qi, or energy, is considered a part of a normal person's health according to traditional Chinese medicine. Having a positive flow of your qi will help your body remain in balance, along with your mind and your emotions.

How Is It Used?

Qigong is used to treat a wide variety of illnesses and conditions. By focusing on one's qi, it is said to open up a positive energy flow in one's body. Conditions such as cancer, depression, and other diseases are said to be cured using this ancient form of medicine.

Qigong healing may be done by a qigong healer, or you can learn the practice to keep yourself healthy and balanced, by not only keeping energy flowing but also by restoring energy as well.

Medical Qigong

As time goes on, this practice has become more widely accepted around the world. In China, it is practiced in hospitals and clinics with astounding results. As the practice gains popularity, it is probable that it will become a part of treatment plans in the United States in the future. While Western medicine is still resistant to these practices, science backs up their results, making it an acceptable form of treatment. We'll talk about qigong in more detail in a later chapter in part 4.

ENERGY MEDICINE AND SCIENCE

In our Westernized society, we are highly reliant on science and its results to tell us whether or not something works. So, you are probably wondering if the practice of energy medicine is scientifically acceptable. For most, the answer is yes. There have been many scientific studies where the practices of energy medicine have been proven to be an acceptable form of treatment for those who are suffering from pain and illness.

While the results are not for everyone, it has been found that the methods behind energy medicine are safer and more effective than some forms of Western medicine. Before taking medications, it might be a great idea to try energy medicine and homeopathic methods to see if they work!

POINTS TO REMEMBER

By going to the source of the problem, energy medicine has been proven to treat illness and disease in a more holistic way than symptom suppression. Homeopathic medicine, Bach flower remedies, acupuncture, and the practice of qigong are just a few of the energy medicine techniques that are practiced around the world.

Scientific results have proven that this indeed is an acceptable method for treating illness and disease and easing pain and discomfort. As time goes by, the Western world is becoming more and more open minded to these practices, which will make them an alternative form of treatment in the future. While the results are great for many, they may not be for everyone. Western medicine still has its place, so don't discount it completely.

We have all heard the saying that "mind over matter" is often the cause of problems. If we can use our mind and body to heal itself, then why not allow this to happen? Energy medicine focuses on this concept. You can essentially heal your own body by using your body's energy and your mind.

Taking the time to explore alternative forms of treatment can open up avenues that you may not have known to exist. I encourage you to keep an open mind and be willing to try alternative methods. You never know, you may find a great way to solve your health problems and live disease free!

REFERENCES FOR CHAPTER 12

Adamson, Wendy. "The Healing Power of Energy Medicine." *Singular Magazine,* June 28, 2015. http://singularcity.com/energy-medicine/ (accessed May 4, 2017).

Bhatia, Manish. "What Is Homeopathy? ABC of Homeopathic Medicine." *Hpathy Ezine,* April 2007. http://hpathy.com/abc-homeopathy/what-is-homeopathy-2/ (accessed May 4, 2017).

Eden, Donna. "Donna Eden Quotes." www.goodreads.com/author/quotes/18158.Donna_Eden.

———. "Quotes by Donna Eden." July 2, 2013. www.awaken.com/2013/07/quotes-by-donna-eden/ (accessed May 4, 2017).

TheFreeDictionary. "Qigong." http://medical-dictionary.thefreedictionary.com/Qigong (accessed May 4, 2017).

HealthWise. "Homeopathy: Topic Overview." *WedMD.* www.webmd.com/balance/guide/homeopathy-topic-overview (accessed May 4, 2017).

Landsman, Jonathan. "Proof That Energy Medicine Works." *Natural News,* January 9, 2014. www.naturalnews.com/043445_energy_medicine_scientific_evidence_Mark_Mincolla.html (accessed May 4, 2017).

National Center for Homeopathy. "What Is Homeopathy?" www.homeopathycenter.org/ (accessed May 4, 2017).

Rogers, Tom. "Qigong: Energy Medicine for the New Millennium." 2004. http://qigonginstitute.org/docs/QigongEMedicine.pdf (accessed May 4, 2017).

Sands, Áine. "Science: Behind the Magic." *Wake Up World,* January 16, 2016. http://wakeup-world.com/2016/01/17/science-behind-the-magic (accessed May 4, 2017).

Singh Deutsch, Dharam. "What Is Medical Qigong?" The Center for Energy Medicine. http://masterhealerdoctor.com/what-is-medical-qigong/ (accessed May 4, 2017).

The Society of Homeopaths. "About Homeopathy?" www.homeopathy-soh.org/about-homeopathy (accessed June 1, 2017).

Stossel, Rich. "New Study Indicates Aging May Be All in Your Head." *Natural News,* May 6, 2013. www.naturalnews.com/040336_aging_longevity_secrets_chi-gung_training.html (accessed May 4, 2017).

Tesla, Nikola. "Nikola Tesla Quotes." www.goodreads.com/author/quotes/278.Nikola_Tesla (accessed May 4, 2017).

Whitaker, Julian. "Homeopathic Remedies: Do They Work?" Dr. Whitaker, December 3, 2014. www.drwhitaker.com/homeopathic-remedies-do-they-work/ (accessed May 4, 2017).

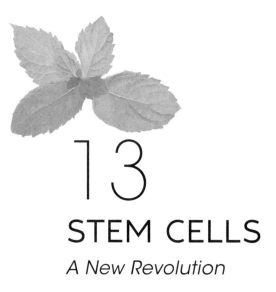

13

STEM CELLS
A New Revolution

Science has presented us with a hope called stem-cell research, which may provide our scientists with answers that have so long been beyond our grasp.

NANCY REAGAN

What can we envision in a future with stem cells? The blind will see, the deaf will hear, and the sick will be cured. Soon, we will live in a world where we will no longer reject our old, aging bodies—a world where we will heal from within.

I want to introduce you to a series of medical treatments that won't saturate your body with drugs or cut it open. Stem-cell treatments include stem-cell injections, intravenous stem-cell solutions, stem-cell transplants, and 3-D-printed stem-cell parts. Regenerative medicine—and stem-cell treatments in particular—relies on the principle that we literally have everything we need in our own bodies to restore and maintain our health. Stem-cell treatments lie at the core of regenerative medicine. After all, what is more regenerative than printing a custom-molded trachea or regenerating a limb using our own stem cells?

In the very near future, people will say, "Can you imagine that they used to open people up? Can you believe they would cut people with scalpels and anesthesia, when they could have easily fixed the problem with a stem-cell injection?" They'll be saying, "Can you believe they gave patients other people's hearts, and livers, and kidneys?"

Stem-cell therapy will become an institution of its own.

Doctors who are smart and forward thinking, who genuinely want to *heal* their patients, will definitely head in this direction. I can see entire practices moving toward preventive and regenerational care, rather than the current modality of symptom suppression and pain management. Stem-cell treatment will become an institution of its own; it will soon become the mainstream in health care. There is no limit to the miraculous results of stem-cell treatments. Continuing research and results will generate more support and funding for stem-cell technologies, ultimately providing care and healing to patients at an affordable cost.

STEM-CELL THERAPY

Stem cells are specialized cells found in the body that can develop into specific cells belonging to a particular organ or part of the body. When we are born, the zygote, which is the single cell formed when an egg is fertilized by a sperm, divides into 150 to 200 embryonic stem cells. This mass of stem cells is known as a blastocyst, and all of the cells found in our body, be it skin cells, blood cells, or brain cells, are formed from this handful of stem cells.

Stem cells are found in adults as well. One well-known example is stem cells found in the bone marrow, which can develop into red blood cells, white blood cells, or platelets. Adult stem cells (also known as tissue-specific stem cells) help in the development and repair and maintenance of the body.

Both embryonic and adult stem cells have two properties that make them so beneficial; they can self-replicate, and they can develop into other types of cells needed by the different organs in the body. Embryonic stem cells are pluripotent, which means they can turn into any type of cell found in the human body, while adult stem cells are multipotent, which means that they can turn into a few types of specific cells that are required for that particular organ or body part.

Stem cell therapy is the use of stem cells in regenerative medicine. Since they can turn into specific cells that the body needs, theoretically, they can be used to cure almost all diseases.

THE SOLUTION WE NEED

As a patient, the worst feeling in the world is despair. You've tried everything. You've gone to every doctor, and they all tell you the same thing: there's nothing more they can do. You've endured every treatment, taken every pill they've prescribed, felt every moment of blinding pain or haunting numbness, and there's nothing left to do.

There are people out there that I personally know who are losing their eyesight or are crippled. They are suffering. They've lost a hip because of prescribed steroid treatments for their chronic asthma. It seems that patients who don't get Alzheimer's get Parkinson's.

These days, you go into a doctor's office, and in three minutes, they look you up and down, and they give you a prescription. Never mind that you're crying because you're in such acute pain, or trying to explain the details of your particular condition and case history. It seems like all they ever say is, "Here, take this prescription."

I want to ignite people out of their complacency.

I want to tell you about the paradigm revolution that is currently taking place, that would completely turn your life around if you gave it a chance. The old paradigm is to go to the doctor when you're already sick, and let the doctor be in charge and call the shots. The new paradigm is when you can visit a number of health care practitioners *while you're still healthy*—when you practice preventive medicine instead of stifling illnesses that you're already suffering from, being much more accountable for your health. It is absolutely essential to take responsibility for your own body and your own life.

At some point in your life, you may feel like you've tried absolutely everything there is to cure yourself of your particular ailment, whether it be achy joints, bulging discs, or chronic heart problems. You may have consulted an orthopedist, and you may have been told that surgery is the only option remaining. But I want to tell you that that's simply not true. Stem-cell treatments are minimally invasive, low risk, and fully capable of repairing and restoring damaged tissue.

Stem-cell injections enable the body to absorb the new, healthy cells in problem areas—knees, hips, even the heart—to promote rejuvenation. By informing ourselves of the possibilities, we can allow stem cells to regenerate our bodies at the cellular level, making us whole again.

Stem-cell treatments will soon be widely available, accessible, and affordable. They will be customized to treat our own specific needs, and they will be the only treatments tailored to our individual bodies.

> **Stem-cell treatments will soon be widely available, accessible, and affordable.**

I am very compassionate about people who are suffering around me. I see my job as an educator and dispeller of ignorance. Ignorance leads many patients to suffer unnecessarily. There are some people with an "old-school mentality," who will not avail themselves of the opportunities out there. They'll just say to me, "Oh, my doctor said to take this medication, and that medication," and all the while, they're still suffering. They have, for years, continued suffering with no end in sight. I see this on a daily basis, and it really breaks my heart.

The only downside to the whole process is that it isn't quite affordable right now. It's not impossible—knee and hip replacements go from $15,000 to $30,000 depending on the extent and location of the hospital, whereas stem-cell treatments cost generally $5,000 and up for a single injection. The biggest and only real drawback is that stem-cell treatments aren't generally covered by insurance, whereas surgeries are, which is why many people would opt to get their "free" surgery. But the benefits of stem-cell treatments definitely outweigh the comparatively brutal surgical procedures, and the cost will definitely decrease as the treatment grows established and widespread.

I want to dissuade you from unnecessary, high-risk surgery.

I want to dissuade you from taking the surgical route *just because* it's covered by your insurance. You may not be paying money for the procedure, but you may be paying very heavily in other ways. There's always a risk when you receive surgery. There's certainly a lot to lose by receiving general anesthesia during these substantial surgical procedures, especially as patient age increases. Many times, people who have hip or knee replacement surgery in their 70s, 80s, or 90s don't ever come back. The anesthesia often deprives the brain of oxygen, with severe consequences. Some patients may lose their memory for good. Others die on the table. Any time there's major surgery, there's always a risk that you can die.

I had a patient who was a smoker, and she was a professional woman who was concerned that everybody was always looking younger. So she went to Chicago to visit the same doctor who did her face, to do her eyes. We had an appointment set up that she missed, so I called her up at home, and when I spoke to her relatives, they told me that she had died during the procedure, while she had been anesthetized. I was shocked, I really was—I had spoken to her only the week before.

You have to be in charge of your own condition, of your own body.

Of course, there may be patients and readers who are resistant to the idea of taking charge of their health. My neighbor is crippled from bulging discs, and he's going to have to go to Arizona now to receive surgery. He could be receiving a stem-cell injection, but he'll be going to Arizona no matter what I say. I'll ask, "What kind of tests have you taken?" or "What do you know about your condition?" He'll say, "I don't know, my doctor has the tests." I'll ask, "What were you high in, and what were you low in?" and he'll say, "Well, I don't know. My doctor said everything was fine." You have to be in charge of your own condition, of your own body. Think for yourself. Consider all the options. Find out what works best for you.

"I've tried *everything*. Enough is enough."

I will provide all the descriptions and examples, all the information you need—but ultimately, it's up to you to choose which path to take. If you're looking into alternative medicine, you've probably encountered a point in your illness and pain when you've thrown up your hands and said, "I've tried everything," or "Enough is enough."

I want to appeal to those of you who wonder, "What if there was something out there that could truly restore my health? That wouldn't just take the pain away, but would bring wholesome healing?" I want you to learn about the option that is less invasive, less risky, and more comprehensive in its healing capacity.

STEM-CELL PROCEDURES: HARVESTING, DEPLOYING, HEALING

Stem cells are wonderfully versatile organisms. We all begin in life as a bundle of stem cells in the womb, each cell taking on a different shape and function. Blood, bone, skin, cartilage—it all begins with stem cells. Then, as we grow up and develop, our bodies activate their natural capacities for healing and regeneration, so that whether we break a bone or have to fight off a cold, our bodies can use a combination of the immune system and naturally generated stem cells to recover.

Stem-cell treatments deploy stem cells where we need them most.

However, as we age, we steadily deplete our supply of stem cells. Our bodies begin to slow down, and we are not able to heal as efficiently, leading to chronic and painful conditions like arthritis, bulging discs, heart disease, and more. Stem-cell treatments tackle this problem by harvesting stem cells from our own bodies and deploying them strategically according to our needs, whether locally through injections, or more generally throughout our bodies using IV (intravenous, or through the bloodstream) solutions. Stem-cell treatments will enable us to recover our natural regenerative capacities, allowing our bodies to heal even as we grow older.

If you feel like you've tried just about everything in traditional medicine, and you're still unsatisfied with the results you've received, you will definitely want to look into the impressive healing potential of stem-cell treatments. You can make an informed decision about whether stem-cell treatments are right for you by contacting a stem-cell practitioner for a consultation. In this section of the book, I will explain the step-by-step procedures of current stem-cell treatments, and I will also introduce two renowned stem-cell institutions in California: the Whitaker Wellness Institute in Newport Beach, and the Irvine Stem Cell Treatment Center in Irvine.

Generally speaking, stem-cell practitioners will follow an order of applications to ensure that they are not overtreating your condition. (An example of overtreatment is using an entire gauze bandage for a tiny paper cut: the treatment doesn't fit the condition, both physically and financially.) A stem-cell treatment, although much simpler than the majority of surgeries, does require liposuction, centrifugation, and deployment, and is therefore left as the last measure.

A respectable orthopedic surgeon may begin your procedure with a series of three cortisone injections over three weeks, a common steroid treatment for joint pain and inflammation. The surgeon will assess your body's reaction to this treatment and check for signs of improvement. If unsatisfactory, the next treatment may be platelet-rich plasma (PRP) injections, which requires the surgeon to draw a sample of your blood and concentrate the plasma count in a centrifuge, promoting greater healing in soft tissues, tendons, ligaments, and joints. Generally, PRP injections have a high rate of success and have even been used satisfactorily in athletic treatment regimes. However, if your condition is severe and beyond the healing capacity of PRP injections, then and only then would a stem-cell practitioner turn to stem-cell injections and IV solutions.

Different institutions may follow different practices of harvesting and deploying stem cells, although the procedures will follow the same general principles. First, the practitioner will perform a minor localized liposuction on the patient, to gain a satisfactory sample of fat cells. This is because fat cells are a rich, easily accessible source of stem cells. Then, the practitioner will process the fat sample through a centrifuge, extracting the stem cells and other regenerative materials. Once the stem cells are isolated, they can be deployed into the body in a number of ways: through injury-specific local injections, like in the spinal column and problematic joints; through the blood stream in an IV solution; or in some cases, in a 3-D printed stem-cell mold to develop into the necessary parts.

When stem cells are deployed directly into the body, they will adapt and take on the form of their surrounding cells, replacing and regenerating over the problematic damaged or worn cells. However, when stem cells are used for developing parts externally, they are inserted into a mold with a sample of the patient's desired body part, whether it be the shell of an ear, a tracheal windpipe, or even a complete human bladder.

At the moment, 3-D printed stem-cell parts are still in the research and development stage, although there have been a number of successful case studies (which I will explore in the coming section). However, stem-cell injections and IV solutions are currently supported by Dr. Whitaker's Wellness Institute, as well as the Irvine Stem Cell Treatment Center.

The Whitaker Wellness Institute

Dr. Whitaker's Wellness Institute specializes in joint restoration in the problem areas of the knee, hip, and spine. The institute uses the latest stem-cell technology to harvest stem cells from the patient's own body. A few ounces of fat—the richest repository of stem cells in adults—are removed during a quick liposuction procedure. Then the fat cells are processed and separated, leaving millions of viable stem cells to be reinjected into the body, wherever the body needs it—locally, at the knee or hip, or intravenously, for respiratory, autoimmune, and neurological conditions. The entire process takes no more than an hour, under local anesthesia and light sedation.

> **The Wellness Institute uses the latest stem-cell technology.**

Dr. Whitaker's Wellness Institute also provides PRP injections, which have successfully treated elite athletes like Kobe Bryant, Tiger Woods, and Peyton Manning and have been brought into the public eye. It's a beneficial therapy for anyone with joint pain caused by injury, overuse, or arthritis.

The Irvine Stem Cell Treatment Center

The Irvine Stem Cell Treatment Center is a renowned Institutional Review Board–based stem-cell therapy network in the United States that also derives and deploys stem cells from fat-transfer technology. Conditions treated by the Irvine Stem Cell Treatment Center include derivative diseases following heart disease, like post myocardial infarction, congestive heart failure, cardiomyopathy, chronic obstructive pulmonary disease; respiratory diseases, like chronic bronchitis, emphysema, and asthma; and neurological conditions, like stroke, Parkinson's disease, cognitive impairment, peripheral neuropathy, multiple sclerosis, and muscular dystrophy.

The center's technology isolates high numbers of viable stem cells.

The center's technology allows them to isolate high numbers of viable stem cells that they can deploy in the same surgical setting—within the same hour, in fact—as the miniliposuction procedure. These stem cells can be deployed either by local injection into the problem area (knee, hip, spine); by IV infusion directly into the patient's bloodstream; or injected directly under the skin.

The Irvine Stem Cell Treatment Center guarantees *no mixing* of cells between patients: all the cells injected into patients at any time are 100 percent their own, which means that there is zero risk for cross-contamination or spread of disease from patient to patient. This process is *even safer* than hospital-standard blood transfusions, because all the components involved are both biologically compatible, and originate completely from the patient's own body. Additionally, their procedure uses a world-tested, sterile "closed system" technology, in which the cells never come into contact with the outside environment, that yields extremely high numbers of viable stem cells.

PROGRESS IN STEM-CELL RESEARCH

The story of the immortal jellyfish became widely publicized in the *New York Times* in 2012, but the jellyfish's ability to restore itself to a juvenile state was first discovered in the 1990s. At the time, the discovery of the jellyfish captivated its researchers: no one knew how its capacity of regeneration could be incorporated into human medicine, but the potential of its powers—its ability to transdifferentiate, or revert its normal body cells into stem cells brimming with potential—seemed absolutely limitless.

> **The immortal jellyfish can naturally transdifferentiate, or revert its body cells back into stem cells.**

The immortal jellyfish marks the beginnings of regenerative medicine, but researchers are pushing for breakthroughs in stem-cell research, both in laboratory and clinical settings. In the current era of technological expansion, countries all over the world are working around the clock to develop safe, efficient methods of harvesting and deploying stem cells into the human body to ensure low-risk, wholesome regeneration. With the rising availability of stem-cell treatments, we are well on our way to a future where we *supply ourselves* with a cache of skin cells, tendons, bones, and even organs.

Here are some recent developments in stem-cell research and case studies that have already begun to make waves in the media.

2006—Lee Spievack: Regenerated Fingertip

Lee Spievack was working on his beloved hobby-shop airplane when, like a scene from a horror movie, the propeller blades suddenly began to spin and took off the tip of his finger. With his finger spurting blood, Lee hurriedly contacted his brother Allen Spievack, a medical researcher, hoping to God that his finger wasn't gone for good. Allen sent over a powdered extract that his team had been working on for some time—a substance called *extracellular matrix* that they had derived from a biological component of pigs' bladders.

> **Lee's finger was completely restored: flesh, bone, and nail.**

Lee didn't know what to expect, but he was desperate to try anything that would help, so he applied the extract and kept his finger tightly wrapped under a gauze bandage. For weeks he waited, and waited. On the day he finally unwrapped his finger, Lee was utterly shocked to see that his finger was completely restored: flesh, bone, and nail. It wasn't a stump. It wasn't a mangled mess of scabs and nail shards. Everything was there, good as new.

2011—Isaias Hernandez: Regenerated Leg Muscles

When the U.S. military heard the news of Lee Spievack's regrown finger, they invested over $70 million dollars into extracellular matrix research, and provided cutting-edge regenerative treatments to veterans all over the nation. So when Isaias Hernandez was hit by an enemy mortar in Afghanistan, the military provided the funding for Isaias to receive injections of extracellular matrix into what remained of his tattered leg muscles.

Now in 2009, Dr. Steven Badylak of the McGowan Institute had suggested that growing entire limbs was only possible "in theory." But in just two years' time between his statement and Isaias's injury, the same extracellular matrix that healed Lee Spievak's finger helped the young marine soldier to regenerate his mutilated leg. The doctors had initially concluded that Isaias's leg *had* to be amputated to prevent infection and risk to his life. But amputation would render Isaias a permanent cripple, which he wasn't prepared to accept. So, under the military-funded regenerative treatment, Isaias found his leg—and his life—fully restored.

2004—Dr. Anthony Atala: 3-D Printed Stem-Cell Organs

Let's go back to the beginnings of the groundbreaking research. Researchers had already managed to grow human organs in animals such as pigs. These animals are called chimeras after the mythological creature that had features of multiple animals. At Wake Forest University in North Carolina, Dr. Anthony Atala was the first to create a functional human stem-cell bladder in a laboratory setting, completely independent of a body. With his team, Dr. Atala has also created muscles, organs, heart valves, and more, adding up to almost twenty different types of functional stem-cell tissues—and this, nearly a decade ago. Dr. Atala explained that we each have a natural store of stem cells in our bodies at any given moment, and they simply need to be prodded into activity to invoke our natural capacity for regenerative healing.

> **Dr. Atala has artificially created muscles, organs, heart valves, and more.**

Medical researchers including Dr. Atala have already successfully transplanted artificially generated organs into mice and sheep, and are currently working on transplanting functioning human bladders. Imagine the possibilities: patients who wait endlessly on organ donor lists can finally look forward to customized stem-cell organs *printed from their own cells.* There are around 120,000 Americans on the transplant list and very few donors. Every day about thirty people die because they can't get a transplant. Organs grown using stem-cell therapy can help reduce this gap and save thousands of lives. Everyone who receives these stem-cell organs will gain a second chance at life and vitality.

2012—Dr. Nabil Dib: Stem-Cell Blood Vessels

Organs aren't the only parts of the body that can—and will—be 3-D printed. At St. John's Regional Medical Center in Oxnard, California, as well as forty-nine additional hospitals, Dr. Nabil Dib and his colleagues have begun isolating adult stem cells to create bioengineered blood vessels. Dr. Dib hopes to use these vessels to create alternative pathways for blood flow, sidestepping the clogged arteries that cause heart disease, heart attacks, and strokes in the body. Not only will the body's stem cells produce these biological bypasses, but the stem cells will also run intravenously (through the blood) to repair the fatigued and failing heart muscles that have strained under years of high-pressure pumping.

> **Dr. Dib hopes to create alternative blood flow using stem-cell blood vessels.**

The stem-cell vessels will lessen patients' need for expensive and high-risk treatments like heart transplants; continued hospitalization; and reduce patients' likelihood of heart failure and death. The treatment will prove to be especially effective for heart attack survivors who haven't responded well to other treatments.

2013—Mel Hudman: Regenerated Hip

The constant pain in Mel's hip kept him from enjoying many aspects of his everyday life. Whether he was limping from place to place or sitting and lying still, his ever-inflamed hip ached and throbbed. The doctors said that there wasn't any cartilage left in his hip to buffer his bones, and the constant grinding pinched his nerves and caused him grief with no end in sight.

Mel had tried everything—chiropractors, reduced movement in a wheelchair, anti-inflammatory pills, you name it. At the end of the line, his doctors recommended a complete hip replacement, which would require six months of rehabilitation, and would not guarantee a painless life.

> **In six months, Mel was able to sit, stand, walk,**
> **and sleep without pain.**

In response, Mel turned to the Whitaker Wellness Institute at the suggestion of his father-in-law. In July 2013, he went to California to receive the institute's renowned stem-cell procedure, which harvested stem cells from a sample of his liposuctioned fat, and injected the cells directly into the hip joint. Within six months—the same recovery time as the hip replacement—Mel was able to sit, stand, walk, and sleep without any pain whatsoever. He finally lives a normal, happy life, freed from his constant burden of pain.

2013—Molly Stevens, Ph.D.: Hybridism and Biomaterial Enhancement of the Body

In a 2013 TED Talk, Molly Stevens, Ph.D., presented her research on bio-materials, or artificial materials (like polymer plastics) that are biologically compatible with the human body. She explained that the technology of biomaterials actually traced back to the days of the ancient Maya, when a lost tooth would be replaced with a piece of blue shell. Although the blue shell was technically a foreign body, the chemical component and architecture of the shell matched human teeth so closely that the gums would cement the blue tooth in place.

Stevens also presented the case study of fighter pilots whose eyes had absorbed bits of plastic that had broken off the shells of planes at high speeds. The researchers were fascinated by the fact that the body did not react *against* the foreign material with inflammation and pain, as is often the case; but rather *absorbed* the material, because it happened to be a material that was biologically compatible with the human body. This same plastic is now being used to create an intraocular lens—a lens that can be inserted directly *into* the eye—to treat cataracts and other types of vision impairments.

> **Stevens's team strives to meet the need for regenerative bone repair.**

Stevens's team has worked extensively to meet the tremendous need for a more wholesome, less painful method of regenerative bone repair. Those suffering from conditions like osteoporosis and fractured bones may face a stem-cell treatment that requires extraction of bone-generated stem cells called the iliac crest graft, which must be harvested from the hip. Although the treatment does allow patients to recover from severe bone fractures and breaks that are beyond natural repair, the harvesting process is often incredibly painful and limited: often, there is not enough iliac crest graft to supply multiple procedures in short succession.

To solve this problem, Stevens's team has developed the "in vivo bioreactor," which prompts the long bones of a leg to regenerate bone material indefinitely. Injecting a specially concocted saline solution under a thin layer of stem cells (the periosteum) along the bones will simultaneously lift the layer from the bone, enabling easier harvesting; but will also create a structured cavity in which the bone can regenerate another layer of bone-generated stem cells. The harvested bone structure has proven to be practically indistinguishable from its original counterpart, potentially providing a means by which to generate massive amounts of bone-patching stem cells.

2014—Acid Bath Treatment: Improved Stem-Cell Production

Researchers around the world were shocked to discover that soaking the blood of newborn mice in a mildly acidic solution could revert the blood cells to their previous stem-cell form. The near-fatal shock of the thirty-minute acid bath creates the pluripotent stem cells that are capable of developing into any type of cell in the body—similar in behavior to the cells of the immortal jellyfish.

> **Blindness, heart disease, muscular dystrophy—these conditions can be remedied with stem-cell treatments.**

Researchers used the principle that stem cells naturally adapt to their surroundings, and successfully multiplied and developed the stem cells into heart, bone, brain, and organ cells by exposing them to cells of the desired material. If this acid bath also worked with human blood cells, it could mean a significant improvement in stem-cell production, which until now has hampered the prevalence of stem-cell treatments.

Although researchers have grown confident about the safe regenerative capacity of stem cells, they have remained at a loss for a biologically efficient and cost-effective supply of stem cells to provide to patients—until now. If researchers establish this method as a legitimate, renewable source of stem cells, any number of medical conditions—including spinal cord injuries, blindness, heart disease, and muscular dystrophy—could be remedied with stem-cell treatments.

There is no longer a space for the one-size-fits-all approach to health care. The biggest complication in medical treatment is that each individual patient is, in fact, individual and unique. Therefore, healing patients with their own stem cells, and in fact their own DNA, reduces the risk of autoimmune rejection; of cross-patient contamination and infection (as is the case with blood transfusions and organ transplants); of harsh and unforeseen side effects from foreign bodies; and ultimately provides an unmatched capacity for full restoration.

2014—Garrett Peterson: 3-D Printed Trachea Transplant for Collapsed Airway

Infant Garrett Peterson received the latest device in 3-D printed, biologically compatible technology. From the moment of his birth, Garrett found it impossible to breathe independently. Severe tracheobronchomalacia softened his trachea and bronchi, collapsing his airways into small slits. To his parents' anguish, Garrett would turn blue four to five times a day, suffering immeasurably from insufficient oxygen. His parents could only watch from the other side of the glass, feeling helpless, frustrated, and desperate.

**Garrett would turn blue four to five times a day,
unable to breathe oxygen.**

Out of options, Garrett's parents turned to the University of Michigan, where associate professor Glenn Green, M.D., and professor Scott Hollister, Ph.D., had created and successfully transplanted a 3-D device that had saved the life of another infant in May 2013. Hollister and Green created a tracheal cast from a biopolymer (biologically compatible plastic) called polycaprolactone that propped open Garrett's airways, so that he was finally able to breathe independently of the machine. They used high-resolution imaging from Garrett's CT scans to produce this biologically compatible structure that would continue to support Garrett's trachea until he no longer needed it, at which point his body would absorb the splint entirely. This would mean that the infant could also avoid any additional surgery to remove the outgrown splint later on.

The biopolymer casts were sewn around Garrett's right and left bronchi to expand the airways and provide external support to aid proper growth. Hollister says that Garrett may need two to three years for his trachea to remodel and grow into a healthier state, which matches the time that his body will take to absorb the biopolymer.

2014—Dr. Wenchun Qu: Stem Cells Restore Spinal Disc Height and Lubrication

Dr. Wenchun Qu of the Mayo Clinic developed a study that recorded the regenerative capacities of stem-cell transplants in reversing degenerative disc disease, or bulging discs. Dr. Qu and his team found that the stem-cell treatments produced a staggering 23.6 percent increase in disc height, indicating the wholesome regeneration of damaged and shattered discs across all six of the groups studied.

**Stem-cell treatments restored spinal discs and lubricant fluids,
reducing friction and pain.**

They also found that the stem-cell transplant increased disc water content, which lubricates and cushions the vertebrae, preventing the painful grinding and pinching that cripples its victims. The stem-cell treatments critically restored the nucleus pulposus structure, or the jellylike substance in the disc, as well as water content in the patients' spines, providing the cushion for the spinal column that would ultimately rid the patients of pain, stiffness, and spinal inflammation.

This was a remarkable breakthrough in the wide range of stem-cell treatments, because current treatments for bulging discs do not counteract the loss of cells and cellular functions. Contrarily, many invasive treatments actually *damage* the disc, causing further degeneration.

2014—Peter Nygard: Restored Vitality

Billionaire fashion designer Peter Nygard has received a record number of stem cell treatments, with reported success. At seventy years old, Nygard has been receiving stem-cell treatments for four years under the close observation of the University of Miami. His treatments were based on the discoveries of Harvard scientists who had successfully regenerated cells in mice and effectively turned back the clock.

Although Nygard appears to be enjoying the renewed prime of his life in his ten-minute YouTube feature, he has stated that the true inspiration for supporting stem-cell research was his mother, whom he had loved very much, and who recently passed away.

Nygard has announced his plans to open a $50 million stem-cell clinic in the Bahamas. With additional research and funding, stem-cell treatments may develop sufficiently to enter the international market at an affordable price, on par with traditional medical treatments.

But practically, scientists are still only learning how to use stem cells for curing a specific disease. The following problems need to be solved in stem-cell research:

- How to ensure that the stem cells develop into exactly those cells that the body needs and not into unwanted cells. If they develop into unwanted cells they can create tumors and even cancer.
- To ensure that the body accepts the stem cells and the immune system does not attack them as foreign bodies.

- Some stem-cell research that was successful in a petri dish might not be successful in animal trials and the success of animal trials might not be replicated in human trials.
- How to obtain stem cells in an ethical and moral way. Religious groups have opposed embryonic stem-cell research because the human blastocyst is destroyed when the embryonic stem cells are obtained.

Stem-cell procedures apply to every and any part of the body. This includes teeth and dental implants; eye and corneal regeneration; rapid treatment of skin grafts; and of course, fingertips. But why stop there? Why not the entire finger, or the entire arm? There is no limit to the reaches of stem-cell technology, and the first step to moving forward is to let patients know the options that are available to them.

> **Why stop there? Why not an entire finger,
> or an entire arm?**

If you are interested in reading more, Life Extension Foundation is one of the best resources out there: LEF is very generous with its information about nutrition and the latest developments in regenerative medicine. It is very well documented and up-to-date.

POINTS TO REMEMBER

We are living in one of the most exciting times in human history. We have unleashed a technology with unlimited potential. In the future, no one will need operations. Everyone will receive stem-cell injections and turn to regenerative medicine to keep their bodies healthy and whole. We will never look at medicine the same way ever again. Stem cells truly mark the start of a worldwide medical revolution.

Unlocking the secrets behind this bioregenerative technology is like stealing fire from the gods. We will soon have the ability to enhance our lives from within.

If stem-cell research succeeds, there isn't a single person who won't benefit, or know someone who will.

MICHAEL J. FOX

REFERENCES FOR CHAPTER 13

Mayo Clinic. "Stem Cells: What They Are and What They Do." www.mayoclinic.org/tests-procedures/bone-marrow-transplant/in-depth/stem-cells/art-20048117 (accessed May 4, 2017).

NIH Stem Cell Information. "Stem Cell Basics: Introduction." National Institutes of Health. https://stemcells.nih.gov/info/basics/1.htm (accessed May 4, 2017).

NIH Stem Cell Information. "What Are Adult Stem Cells?" National Institutes of Health, February 20, 2008. https://stemcells.nih.gov/info/basics/4.htm (accessed May 4, 2017).

NIH Stem Cell Information. "What Are Embryonic Stem Cells?" National Institutes of Health. https://stemcells.nih.gov/info/basics/3.htm (accessed May 4, 2017).

NIH Stem Cell Information. "What Are the Potential Uses of Human Stem Cells and the Obstacles That Must Be Overcome before These Potential Uses Will Be Realized?" National Institutes of Health, February 20, 2008. https://stemcells.nih.gov/info/basics/7.htm (accessed May 4, 2017).

Robinson, B. A. "Stem Cell Research: All Viewpoints." Religious Tolerance.org. www.religioustolerance.org/res_stem.htm (accessed May 4, 2017).

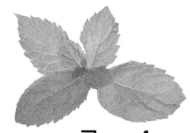

14

EPIGENETICS
Unraveling Your DNA

While weight loss is important, what's more important is the quality of food you put in your body—food is information that quickly changes your metabolism and genes.

MARK HYMAN

When Loretta came to see me in my practice some twenty-five years ago, she was fifty years old and very thin, with hypoglycemia. She was very concerned that she would get breast cancer because her mother was diagnosed with breast cancer when she turned fifty-five and died of the disease. Then at the age of fifty-five, her sister got breast cancer and had a mastectomy.

She told me that she had decided to go on a very low- or no-fat diet (which was the fad at that time, because fat was an estrogen precursor, and estrogen was a promoter of cancer, she told me). You might recall that at that time fat was demonized by everyone, including doctors, the food industry, and dietitians as being unhealthy. Today we know differently. We know there's a difference between good and bad fats. Although she was very thin she continued to consume an enormous amount of sugar, which she craved due to her hypoglycemia.

At the age of fifty-five, Loretta too was diagnosed with breast cancer and had a mastectomy. At that time, the term *epigenetics* wasn't even coined, and the correlation between cancer and sugar was relatively unknown. I can't help but wonder if she had not gone on such an extreme diet that eliminated fat, which actually improves immunity, and eliminated sugar instead, whether she would have even been diagnosed with cancer. As you will see in this chapter, foods, supplements, and lifestyle can not only influence genetic expression, but actually downregulate hereditary disposition.

We are all born with the genes that we inherit from our parents, but how and whether our body expresses these genes is gaining increasing attention in the emerging science of epigenetics. The term *epigenetics* means "on top of the gene." This means that even though we might have a hereditary or genetic predisposition for a certain disease, it is possible to bypass acquiring the illness. Having a gene is not the same as activating a gene. The activation part depends on lifestyle and diet and other factors.

Epigenetics research suggests that maintaining sufficient nutrient levels will significantly affect your current and future health. Keep in mind, it is not only our nutritional level, but also our emotional well-being that can affect how our genes are expressed. For example, a sedentary lifestyle can amplify the effects of a genetic tendency toward obesity, while a daily walk can reduce genetic influence toward obesity. Meditation can also epigenetically influence our genes. Meditation can suppress genes responsible for inflammation and therefore help you physically recover more quickly.

The deeper we delve into this newly growing field of epigenetics, the more reason we find to approach health naturally, through lifestyle modifications and a wholesome diet, dietary supplements, and a positive frame of mind.

In this chapter, we are going to take a look at the role that epigenetics plays in our lives and lifestyles. We will also be examining the role of emotions and how they can alter genetic expression.

WHAT IS EPIGENETICS?

Through studies and other research, it is believed that environmental factors, diet, and other conditions can actually affect the way genes express themselves. We have a lot of genes that stay in the off, or inactivated, state under normal conditions. But outside factors can activate them or deactivate other genes. Some of these epigenetic expressions can be passed down from people to their offspring and even generations down the line from the original person who lived in these conditions.

What does this mean for you? Under the concept of epigenetics, if one of your parents or even grandparents made some not-so-healthy lifestyle choices, you can feel the effects of these decisions. If one of your parents overeats, it might have switched on the obesity gene in their body and they might have passed down this activated gene to you, making it more difficult for you to lose weight.

The next time that someone thinks that his choices only affect his life, tell him that this is a misconception. Your choices can have long-lasting effects not only on your health and longevity, but also the health and longevity of your future descendants.

HOW DOES IT AFFECT ME?

Now that you have a basic understanding of epigenetics, you may be wondering how it pertains to your life. The choices that your grandparents and your parents made are affecting you right now, even though you may not realize the consequences of their choices. Also, the choices that you are making right now can affect your offspring.

> **Your choices can have long-lasting effects
> on your future descendants.**

By understanding epigenetics and the consequences of your actions on the genes that you pass down, you may rethink some of the health choices that you are making right now. If your choices can affect your descendants, then you may want to consider how you live your life and the ways in which you treat your body.

The good news? Epigenetics can also have a positive effect on your life and that of your offspring. The healthy choices that you make right now can be passed down and show their benefits in future generations. Even if you haven't made the best choices, it's never too late to change!

BENEFITS OF EPIGENETICS

While having a basic understanding of epigenetics may help you to change some of your habits, there are other benefits to the concept. By changing your diet and exercise routines, giving up unhealthy habits, and making better choices, you may be preparing yourself for a longer, healthier life. Let's take a look at a few ways that you can benefit your body through the concept of epigenetics.

Fasting

In a study performed at the University of Florida, it was found that intermittent fasting actually benefited the body in several ways. During the study, the test group would alternate fasting days with feasting days. The participants in the study found it easier to fast than to feast.

How is this beneficial to epigenetics? In the fasting state, it is found that free radicals are released and that promotes longevity. Having these free radicals released intermittently helps your body to build up a tolerance for them, making it possible to enhance longevity.

Avoiding GMOs

Just like humans, plants can also be affected by epigenetics. In fact, plants and microbes are much more affected by epigenetics than animals. When plants are modified, the modifications can reach on for generations to come. Since plants are more susceptible to epigenetic influences, it can be harmful to the organism to endure too many genetic changes.

By avoiding GMOs, you are avoiding eating genetically altered foods that can have a negative effect on your own health. While people may believe that the changes made make the organism better, it is really messing with its genetics and can cause problems later on.

Changing Your Mind-Set When It Comes to Health

When it comes to health and pursuing a healthy lifestyle, the way that you view your lifestyle can have a huge effect on how it works in your life. By being positive about how you talk about and perceive your health, you will mentally be putting yourself on that path. Have you ever heard the term "mind over matter"? This term speaks volumes when it comes to how you feel. If you tell yourself that you are happy and feeling good, you are more likely to feel that way. If you are constantly focusing on how bad you feel, you will feel bad more often.

By knowing and understanding what your body is telling you and what your family history tells you, you can mentally prepare yourself for whatever may be in your future. Your mind is a powerful tool for your health and your well-being. How you perceive yourself and your health can have a huge impact on how healthy and happy you really are.

IMPROVING YOUR LONGEVITY
THROUGH EPIGENETICS

Changing your diet and exercise habits now can actually help you boost your longevity. While you may not have had the best habits in the past, making an effort to improve these habits can have lasting benefits for your future. Knowing and understanding your health risks and how to avoid them can help you to live a longer and healthier life.

What epigenetics does is show that your life is really in your own hands. Sure, you might be suffering from some bad decisions made by your parents or grandparents but you still have the ultimate control over your gene expression. Making healthy lifestyle choices can actively alter your gene expression and it will help you to improve your longevity. And your future generations will also be thankful to you.

GUIDING YOUR GENE EXPRESSION

Knowing that you can ultimately change the course of your life and the lives of your offspring can be a great motivator for changing possibly damaging habits. By making healthy and proactive changes now, you can change your gene expression and that of your children and even grandchildren. As a parent, you want the best for your children, right? Start with focusing on yourself and the genes that you are passing down to future generations.

> You can change your gene expression, and that of your children, by making healthy proactive choices right now.

Emotions and Gene Expression

For those of you who are easily stressed, epigenetics might just give you a reason to stop the stressing out. It has been proven that your emotions have a link to epigenetics and gene expression. As I mentioned before, "mind over matter" really does play a role in how our genes are read and play out. Our thoughts and feelings can ultimately affect how our genes are read and how they express themselves.

Learning to control your emotions can help promote positive gene expression. Diseases such as cancer can actually be prevented by having positive emotions. Understanding how your mind-set can affect your gene expression might have you trying to change your state of mind.

So think positive thoughts and keep negative emotions in check. It is not bad to feel negative emotions like sadness and anger from time to time. That after all is what it means to be human. But you should not get swept away in these negative emotions. You are the master of your emotions, not the other way around.

The reason why people get stuck in negative emotions is because they try hard to avoid them. This might sound paradoxical but it's true. When we think of negative emotions as bad and try to avoid feeling them at all costs, these negative emotions build up within us. Small sad emotions begin to pile up and one day you find that there is a lot of negative emotion within you and it will actually change your gene expression and make you physically ill.

The way to deal with negative emotions is to feel them fully and then move on. Think of emotions like waves in the sea. The crests of happiness have to be followed by troughs of sadness. Let the emotions flow freely. When you do that, when you allow yourself to feel negative emotions, you'll find that you are happy most of the time and when you do get sad, it always passes. The sadness will actually help you appreciate your happiness even more. You won't build up a huge store of negative emotion and will never feel depressed.

How Your Habits Will Affect Your Children's Genes

You may not be able to change the genes that you have already passed down to your existing children, but by making changes that include your children, you can help end the negative gene expressions that may already exist.

You may have passed on a predisposition for your children to smoke or overeat. However, you can stop smoking and overeating and encourage your children to do the same. It's not too late to try to alter the course that gene expression may take in your offspring.

The Role Your Diet Plays in Gene Expression

Your health and diet can have long-term effects on you and your offspring. If you eat a healthy and balanced diet, then your genes are more likely to express themselves in the way that they were meant to in the beginning. However, if you have an unhealthy diet, it can cause changes in the way in which your genes are read, altering how your body reacts. Having healthy habits now can have lasting effects on how our futures play out.

So eat healthy, eat whole foods, avoid processed foods, and eat in moderation. Do not overeat, and limit your intake of sugar. Eat fresh and organic food and include a lot of vegetables in your diet. Don't just eat muscle meat but also organ meat. By doing all this, you will help your genes express in the right way.

EPIGENETICS AND DISEASE

It has been a belief that cancer is a genetically driven disease. In some cases that is true, but it is also true that cancer can be epigenetically driven. Our lifestyle choices and diet can affect the way in which our genes are read, making cancer a possibility for those who do not necessarily have a genetic predisposition to the disease. Not only cancer, but other supposed genetic illnesses can also be epigenetically driven.

Cancer can be driven by epigenetics.

Are you destined to succumb to disease just because your parents had it? Not necessarily. In the media, we have seen stars such as Angelina Jolie taking measures to prevent breast cancer because her mother had the disease. Even though she has never been diagnosed with breast cancer, she decided to nip the problem in the bud and have a double mastectomy to prevent herself from getting the disease at all. What she doesn't know is that she may have caused herself more harm than good by taking such a dramatic step. Studies have shown that women with a family history of breast cancer are less likely to "inherit" the disease. The environment that you are in will have more influence on the genes than your family history.

While Angelina Jolie's actions were drastic and probably unnecessary, there are other ways that you can protect yourself against diseases. First of all, ensuring that you have a healthy diet and exercise routine are two of the main ways that you can change your gene expression. By eating foods that fight disease, you can limit the likelihood that you will acquire the disease.

Another way that you can help prevent cancer is by upping your intake of curcumin. This nutrient has been proven to be an anticarcinogen, actually fighting the cancer cells already present in your body. Most cancers are not pronounced right away, so fighting the odds of cancer through curcumin can reduce your chances of being diagnosed with the disease. Curcumin can be found in turmeric extract, so look for this when looking for a source of curcumin.

Another supplement that may be useful in changing your genetic expression is DIM (diindolylmethane). DIM is part of a compound that has anticancer properties and is actually very easy to acquire through your diet. This compound can be found in broccoli and cabbage and has been proven to help prevent breast cancer! DIM is found in I3C (indole-3-carbinole). While I3C doesn't last very long in your body, DIM continues to circulate. How does DIM prevent breast cancer? It actually regulates hormone imbalance in the body and influences cell behavior. If you have unbalanced estrogen in your body, DIM is a great way to put it in check!

Benefits of DIM include:

• Blockage of cancer cells
• Preventing metastasis of cancer cells
• Killing cancer cells
• Being effective against several types of cancers

How can this affect you even if you don't have cancer? Start eating your veggies now and help prevent cancer in your future!

CASE STUDY OF EPIGENETICS: THE HOLOCAUST

As the history books tell us, the Holocaust was a tragic time where the Jews were persecuted and punished for their genetic backgrounds. During this period in time, this group of people were picked out, persecuted, and put to death due to their heritage. Taking a look at this group of people can be a useful case study in figuring out how epigenetics can affect a group of people.

A study was conducted where they found thirty-two individuals who had lived during this period of time and experienced the persecution of the Holocaust. Looking at how the stress affected the individuals who experienced the trauma firsthand and how it affected their children gives us a clear picture of how epigenetics can affect offspring and future generations.

By studying the DNA of the children of those who experienced the Holocaust, they found genetic indicators of stress and trauma in the children, even though the children never experienced it themselves. Through the research, they found that certain stress and trauma markers affected the gene expression of the children of Holocaust survivors.

> The children of Holocaust survivors had the same genetic indicators of stress and trauma as their parents, even though they had not gone through the Holocaust themselves.

The research concludes that even though the children of the Holocaust survivors didn't experience the trauma firsthand, they still shared the same fears and stresses as their parents who survived that period. This is clear proof that genes and genetic predisposition to trauma can be passed down from generation to generation.

POINTS TO REMEMBER

Genes are powerful. We get a lot of who we are through the genes that our parents pass along to us. Some of these genes can be wonderful, giving us attributes that we love about ourselves. Other genes may be a detriment to our health and happiness. Your genetic makeup can be affected by your parents and their habits. Your habits can also be passed down to your children through epigenetics.

Gene expression can be influenced by your lifestyle, habits, and emotions. These gene markers can be passed down to your offspring. By making changes toward positive habits now, you can influence your gene expression and that of your offspring for the better. It's not too late to start moving toward the positive side. By taking the time to change your diet, exercise, and how you deal with stressors, you can affect your own longevity, along with the longevity of your children and grandchildren.

Knowing how we can influence our health and that of future generations may make us think more clearly about how we act when it comes to our health. Having the knowledge of epigenetics and gene expression can help us make positive changes right now. What can you change that will help influence your future health and that of your descendants?

REFERENCES FOR CHAPTER 14

ANH-USA. "Epigenetics Also Warns Us about GMOs." Alliance for Natural Health, January 28, 2014. www.anh-usa.org/epigenetics-also-warns-us -about-gmos/ (accessed May 4, 2017).

———. "If You Care about Your Health, You Need to Know about the Emerging Science of Epigenetics." Alliance for Natural Health, January 28, 2014. www .anh-usa.org/science-of-epigenetics/ (accessed May 4, 2017).

Baylor College of Medicine. "Epigenetic Changes Can Drive Cancer, Study Shows." *Science Daily,* July 26, 2014. www.sciencedaily.com/releases/2014 /07/140726082322.htm (accessed May 4, 2017).

Chopra, Deepak. "Mindful Evolution: Can You Guide What Your Genes Are Doing?" *SFGate,* July 21, 2015. www.sfgate.com/opinion/chopra/article /Mindful-Evolution-Can-You-Guide-What-Your-Genes-6391542.php (accessed May 4, 2017).

Church, Dawson. "Kickstarting Your Longevity Genes: The Epigenetic Benefits of Intermittent Fasting." *HuffPost,* September 17, 2015. www .huffingtonpost.com/dawson-church/kickstarting-your-longevi_b_8096262 .html (accessed May 4, 2017).

Dowshen, Steven. "What Is Epigenetics?" *KidsHealth,* January, 2014. http:// kidshealth.org/en/parents/about-epigenetics.html (accessed May 4, 2017).

Landsman, Jonathan. "Emotions Proven to Alter Genetic Expression." *Natural News,* September 5, 2014. www.naturalnews.com/046747_emotions_genetic _expression_physical_health.html (accessed May 4, 2017).

McTaggart, Lynne. "What Doctors Didn't Tell Angelina Jolie." LMct.com, May 31, 2013. http://lynnemctaggart.com/what-doctors-didnt-tell-angelina -jolie-2/ (accessed May 4, 2017).

Mercola, Joseph. "Cancerous Cells Cannot Thrive Without This." *Mercola,* June 13, 2011. http://articles.mercola.com/sites/articles/archive/2011/06/13/this -powerful-herb-changes-your-genes-to-combat-cancer.aspx (accessed May 4, 2017).

———. "You Really Are What You Eat: Your Diet Alters How Your Genes Behave." *Mercola,* February 22, 2016. http://articles.mercola.com/sites /articles/archive/2016/02/22/you-are-what-you-eat.aspx (accessed May 4, 2017).

Minton, Barbara L. "Supplements of DIM Stop Many Cancers in Their Tracks." *Natural News,* March 10, 2009. www.naturalnews.com/025810_cancer _estrogen_cancers.html (accessed May 4, 2017).

Northrup, Christiane. "4 Powerful Ways to Improve Your Health and Longevity with Epigenetics." Christiane Northrup, M.D., June 7, 2015. www.drnorthrup .com/4-powerful-ways-to-improve-your-health-and-longevity-with -epigenetics/ (accessed May 4, 2017).

Thomson, Helen. "Study of Holocaust Survivors Finds Trauma Passed on to Children's Genes." *Guardian,* August 21, 2015. www.theguardian.com/science /2015/aug/21/study-of-holocaust-survivors-finds-trauma-passed-on-to -childrens-genes (accessed May 4, 2017).

The Week. "Epigenetics: How Our Experiences Affect Our Offspring." January 20, 2013. http://theweek.com/articles/468627/epigenetics-how-experiences -affect-offspring (accessed May 4, 2017).

What Doctors Don't Tell You. "Gene Genie." July 2013. www.wddty.com/magazine /2013/july/gene-genie.html (accessed May 4, 2017).

15

CUTTING-EDGE REGENERATIVE TREATMENTS

The best way to predict the future is to create it.

PETER DRUCKER

Regenerative medicine is no longer a dream for the future, it is happening right now. Medical science has made tremendous leaps in recent years, which has brought cutting-edge regenerative treatments into the mainstream. We are also beginning to understand the health benefits of natural substances such as cannabis that have been wrongly grouped with harmful drugs.

In this chapter, we'll discuss such therapies that will be a standard part of medicine in the future. These alternative therapies and futuristic treatments need to be studied and explored so that we can all benefit from them.

Regenerative medicine is happening right now!

PRP THERAPY

PRP, platelet-rich plasma, is prepared by drawing the patient's blood and separating the platelets in a centrifuge. The concentrated platelets are then injected into the patient's body in the location where regenerative healing is required. PRP therapy has recently become popular with top level athletes to heal sports injuries but it has been around since the 1980s.

The platelets in our blood have many functions and the most commonly known function is to form clots to stop bleeding. But platelets also help in healing the body by regenerating cells. PRP therapy can help in recovery from injuries such as tendon or ligament injury, nerve injury, chronic tendonitis, osteoarthritis, bone repair and regeneration, oral surgery and plastic surgery.

PRP therapy is not covered by insurance because there are no large-scale, randomized, double-blind, clinical trials that prove that PRP therapy works. There are smaller trials and some of them have shown promising results but most of the popularity of this therapy comes from anecdotal evidence given by individuals who have used it. The procedure requires thirty minutes to an hour and the prices range from $300 to $1,000 per injection. Ultrasound is used to locate the exact spot where the injection is to be given.

The attraction of PRP therapy is based on the fact that it is a high-end natural therapy. Since the patient's own blood is used, the therapy is completely natural. But it should be remembered that even though it is natural, high concentration of a natural substance can also be harmful. Further trials are needed to ensure the safety of this therapy and to prove its efficacy beyond any doubt.

3-D BIOPRINTING

3-D printing has revolutionized not just the engineering and manufacturing world but also the medical world. It allows for surgeons to print bone components designed specifically for a particular patient. There are many cases where people have received a plastic skull or a titanium jaw or a custom-designed disc for the vertebra. But now 3-D printing has gone one step further by making it possible to print out tissue and even whole organs using biological material. This is known as 3-D bioprinting.

The most common method of 3-D bioprinting is to use an inkjet printer with a bio-ink that is made up of cells and nutrients and a hydrogel to hold everything together. Laser printers and extrusion printers can also be used. 3-D bioprinting has been used to create tissue for testing drugs. Bone, muscle, cartilage, and other types of tissue can all be printed but the major problem used to be the creation of the channels and blood vessels that are necessary for the survival of the tissue as they bring the nutrients and oxygen to the cells. This problem has now been solved using a system called the Integrated Tissue and Organ Printing System (ITOP). This system allows for channels to be printed into the tissue, which allows for the flow of nutrients.

Complete organs are also being printed but scientists are still struggling to keep them alive for a long time. For one thing, organs are complex and they have to be mapped closely using MRI and other scanning techniques to get the exact model for printing.

Next, they need to have the proper tubes and channels for blood and nutrients to flow through them. Also, creating a working organ is not simply a matter of accurately mapping and printing the organ. Say you print out an exact replica of the heart, but how do you get it to run like a heart? Where's the start button? The spark of life happens in a way that scientists still don't understand. But the scientists are continuing research and are getting closer to it.

Already, they've managed to create a functioning liver that stays alive for forty days. The day when your own cells will be used to print a fully functioning organ and every hospital will have an organ printing machine isn't too far away.

> **In the future we will have organs 3-D printed to order.**

HYPERBARIC OXYGEN THERAPY

Hyperbaric oxygen therapy has been around for a long time and in the beginning was used to treat decompression sickness that deep-sea divers can suffer from if they surface from the depths too quickly. It is also cleared as a treatment for certain diseases such as carbon monoxide poisoning, severe anemia, air bubbles in the blood vessels, burns, gangrene, skin infections that kill the tissue, radiation injury, and healing wounds that won't heal easily like diabetic foot ulcer.

It is also used by some private clinics and alternative medicine practitioners to treat other diseases such as cancer, AIDS, Alzheimer's, cerebral palsy, asthma, depression, heatstroke, heart disease, migraine, spinal cord injury, sports injuries, and stroke. However, the FDA has not approved HBOT, as it is often called, as a treatment for these diseases and so insurance does not cover it for them.

Despite the FDA's reluctance to approve HBOT for additional diseases, and the continued stubbornness of mainstream medicine in overlooking the potential of HBOT, many people have achieved great results with this therapy to fight all kinds of diseases and conditions. You can understand its potential when you understand how HBOT works.

Simply put, hyperbaric oxygen therapy increases the amount of oxygen present in the blood of the patient. It can be done in two ways; either by letting the patient inhale 100 percent oxygen from a mask or by increasing the pressure of the room, which effectively increases the oxygen inhaled in each breath. Usually both of these are done together in HBOT. The increased oxygen helps the body to function at full throttle and the body can heal itself faster. It also improves immune function and has an anti-inflammatory effect. Many people, especially if they are sick, suffer from cellular hypoxia, which means that their body isn't getting enough oxygen at the cellular level. This hampers their body's ability to heal itself. HBOT is very useful in such conditions.

There is a fear among some doctors that higher oxygen in the body can result in increased free radicals, which can cause harm to the body. But just like a little exercise is good for you even though it stresses the body, HBOT sessions can actually kick-start the body's immune system by increasing the free radicals for a short while. Unlike other medicines, which can't be undone once the pill is taken, HBOT's effects disappear as soon as the session is over. So it is very safe to try and the kind of oxygen toxicity that the FDA warns about can only occur when very high doses of oxygen are given in a high-pressure chamber.

Mild HBOT can be tried at home by patients by investing in a flexible or portable pressure chamber. Oxygen bottles or an oxygen concentrator can be used along with a pressure chamber to take mild HBOT sessions at a private clinic or even right at home. Athletes often use it not just to heal injuries, but also to recover faster after an event or a workout session. It is even used by racehorse owners to help the horses recover faster between races. Vets use these chambers to help animals recover from surgery.

Other risks involved with this therapy are temporary nearsightedness, middle ear injuries, lung collapse if the pressure changes abruptly, oxygen toxicity, and a risk of fire if a spark is induced in the pressure chamber. But all of these risks are very rare. Oxygen toxicity only happens at very high doses; chances of fire are eliminated by not allowing any flammable objects or objects that might spark inside the pressure chamber. So, there is a lot of advantage in trying out hyperbaric oxygen therapy if you are looking for an alternative regenerative therapy.

HYALURONIC ACID

Paul came to my practice through his doctor's recommendation. He is a long-distance bicycle rider. In fact he and his wife biked around the world. The problem was his knees. Being in his late seventies, he had severe osteo-arthritis of the knees and several doctors recommended knee replacement, which he wanted to avoid.

I had suggested trying hyaluronic acid as a supplement and although it gave him some relief at the time, he was looking for a longer-term solution. I then suggested hyaluronic acid injections; these are sometimes called "rooster comb injections" because of where the substance comes from. He found a doctor who was willing to give him injections and his knees do not bother him anymore. He needs to go in several times per year for booster injections, but is otherwise doing well.

Hyaluronic acid is a substance that is found naturally in the body in connective tissue, neural tissue, and epithelial tissue. It is found in the highest concentration in the eyes and in joints. It is used to treat osteo-arthritis and can be injected directly into the joints or can be taken orally. It is also used to replenish the natural fluids of the eyes during eye surgery such as cataract surgery. As mentioned in chapter 5 on skin, it is also used as a dermal filler by plastic surgeons.

Hyaluronic acid is also said to have healing properties and can be used to heal skin wounds, burned skin, skin ulcers, and dry skin. It is also playing an important role in 3-D bioprinting research. It acts like a biocompatible scaffold that supports the cellular structure of the tissue.

MEDICAL CANNABIS

You might have seen the special on CNN that Dr. Sanjay Gupta did several years back on a little girl with epilepsy who was having so many epileptic seizures per day that she was endangering her life. Her mother had tried all the medications on the market to no avail. She then heard about a form of medical cannabis called CBD that does not produce the "high" of THC (*Cannabis sativa* L-strain with less than 3 percent THC) and found a grower who was willing to supply her child with it. She was given a tincture form orally and her seizures were dramatically reduced to just a few a week. This incident, "Charlotte's Web," completely changed Dr. Sanjay Gupta's mind about medical marijuana, and he began a series of programs about the application of this regenerative treatment on many other kinds of health problems.

Medical cannabis is the new ancient therapy. As more and more research is done around the world on cannabis, more and more benefits of this powerful herb are coming out in the open. This new information is slowly helping it get rid of the bad reputation that cannabis has gotten over the years. The truth is that if used correctly, medical marijuana can be a highly useful form of therapy against a myriad of diseases and conditions.

History of Cannabis

Today, most people imagine a hippie getting stoned when they think of marijuana but actually cannabis has been used in ancient medicine for over 5,000 years. Cannabis has three species; *sativa, indica,* and *ruderalis* and the plant is indigenous to the Indian subcontinent and Central Asia. It was grown as hemp and is supposed to be one of the oldest domesticated crops in the world. Hemp was a wonderful crop that was used for hemp oil, hemp seeds, and hemp fiber to make paper, ropes, and cloth. It was also used in medicine. Hemp is still grown in many countries.

The ancient cultivators selectively bred cannabis to produce the varieties of hemp and marijuana. The major difference between the two is that hemp contains very little THC, the psychoactive substance of marijuana. Hemp plants also are mostly male and do not produce flower buds while marijuana plants are mostly female and produce lots of buds.

The use of cannabis for medical purposes began in China somewhere around 2700 BCE. It spread from China to Asia, the Middle East, and Africa. Cannabis was even used by the Greeks as a medicine. Indian culture has always had a special place for cannabis. It has been used for medical, recreational, religious, and spiritual purposes for thousands of years in India. A papyrus found in Egypt dated back to 1550 BCE notes the use of cannabis for medical purposes. In 200 CE a Chinese surgeon was the first to use cannabis as an anesthetic during surgery. Cannabis was used in the Middle Ages all over the Middle East as hashish. It was used in place of wine, which was banned. It was also used in folk medicine all over Europe.

During the American colonization, hemp was used as a major crop but marijuana was introduced as a psychoactive drug much later.

Endocannabinoid System

Cannabis contains compounds called cannabinoids that have psychoactive and medical properties. Two of the major cannabinoids are THC, or tetrahydrocannabinol, and CBD, or cannabidiol. CBN and CBG are two among many other cannabinoids but their role and benefits aren't as well understood as THC and CBD. The reason why these cannabinoids are so powerful is because our body has built-in receptors for these chemicals.

The human endocannabinoid system has endogenous cannabinoid receptors located in the brain and in the nervous system. Our body naturally produces substances that get attached to these receptors, and when that happens, the body responds by regulating appetite, mood, memory, immune system, and pain sensation. THC and CBD are phytocannabinoids that, when ingested, attach to these receptors and bring about a similar physiological response in the body.

Two main receptors, namely CB1 and CB2, are activated by the cannabinoids. CB1 receptors are mostly found in the brain and the reproductive organs. THC targets CB1 receptors and its most important effect is pain modulation. THC is the one responsible for the psychoactive effects of cannabis.

CB2 receptors are mostly found in the immune system, especially in the spleen. CBD activates this receptor and has an anti-inflammatory response in the body. CBD also moderates the effect of THC by knocking it out of the receptors and taking its place.

This shows that not only does cannabis have beneficial effects for the body, but the body actually produces its own cannabinoids. If the body isn't producing enough endocannabinoids, it makes sense to consume them through medical cannabis to help the body function better.

Benefits of Cannabis
Medical cannabis has the following benefits:

- Helps in mood regulation and fights depression
- Helps in fighting PTSD, anxiety, and other stress-related problems
- CBD oil can be used in medicine to prevent seizures in children— cannabis has been used to fight seizures since 1800 BCE
- Fights multiple sclerosis
- Fights degenerative neurological diseases such as Parkinson's disease
- Fights Alzheimer's disease in multiple ways: decreases amyloid beta production; anti-inflammatory and antioxidant properties of cannabis help prevent the onset of Alzheimer's; protects the neurons from damage due to oxidation; and has been known to promote the growth of new neurons
- Fights cancer in multiple ways: activating the CB1 and CB2 receptors has a cascading effect on the immune system, which helps in maintaining a healthy body; when enough endocannabinoids aren't being produced, cancer can grow; taking cannabinoids through cannabis can help in preventing cancer and can even help in killing off cancer by activating apoptosis or programmed cell death; it can be used to reduce the side effects of chemotherapy such as nausea; and studies have found that cannabis is helpful in brain cancer, breast

cancer, lung cancer, blood cancer, prostate cancer, liver cancer, pancreatic cancer, oral cancer, and colon cancer

- Fights infections and cures diseases such as tuberculosis due to antibacterial properties—it can even work against bacteria that have become resistant to standard antibiotics
- CBD has been known to improve the efficiency of mitochondria of brain cells, which improves brain function
- Increases appetite in patients suffering from malnutrition or appetite loss

Why Is Cannabis Demonized?

If cannabis has so many medical benefits, why has it been demonized in the mainstream media? Marijuana got its bad reputation in the 60s when the psychedelic culture led to selective breeding of cannabis plants to increase the psychoactive THC levels and reduce the CBD levels. A lot of harmful drugs were being used during that era and sadly marijuana was bundled in with the likes of LSD, heroin, and cocaine during Nixon's war on drugs.

> Cannabis has so many benefits and so few harmful effects that it deserves to be studied properly and removed from the list of deadly drugs.

To this day marijuana is considered to be a Schedule 1 drug but it doesn't fit the criteria to be in this group. The drugs in this group should have a high potential for abuse, should have no accepted medical use, and should have a lack of safety even under medical supervision. But marijuana fails all three criteria. It has a very low potential for abuse, it has a lot of medical uses, and it is very safe. The cannabinoid receptors are not present in the areas of the brain that regulate heart rate and respiration so it can't lead to death due to drug overdose.

On top of that, there are varieties of cannabis that have all the medical benefits with very little or no psychoactive effects. The two most common breeds, *indica* and *sativa,* should not be considered identical as they have different levels of THC and CBD. Higher levels of CBD help in fighting the psychoactive and panic-inducing effects of THC.

The problem with this demonization of cannabis is that scientists can't do the research necessary to uncover and prove its medical benefits. So we need to educate the masses about the different types of cannabis and their beneficial uses so that we can look deeper into this magical herb and who knows what new benefits we'll find. It might even be an important key in finding a cure for cancer.

How to Use Medical Cannabis

The good news is that a lot of states have begun to allow the use of medical marijuana in certain cases. You still need to get a prescription from your physician in the form of a medical marijuana card. There are many ways to consume medical marijuana.

Inhalation: It allows for titration of the dosage and has an instantaneous effect.

Smoking: Marijuana can be smoked as a joint mixed in a cigarette, through a pipe, or a bong. Smoking isn't the most effective way of using marijuana as a lot of the healing properties are lost in the smoke. Smoking a joint has all the negative effects of smoking a tobacco cigarette. If you must smoke, the best way is through a bong or a water pipe as the water absorbs some of the harmful materials present in the smoke.

Vaporization: It is a very good way to inhale marijuana and has very few side effects.

Sublingual or oral mucosal: Cannabis oil or tinctures can be used by dropping them in the mouth or below the tongue. This is a good option for people who do not smoke, like children suffering from seizures.

Oral ingestion: Edible cannabis can be added to foods such as cookies, brownies, tea, or in the form of pills. There are certain concerns regarding the absorption of the fat-soluble cannabinoids through this method.

Topical application: Cannabis is available as a lotion or ointment for skin inflammation, muscle pain, and arthritis but it is not understood how the cannabinoids are absorbed through the skin.

POINTS TO REMEMBER

Regenerative techniques like PRP therapy, 3-D printing, HBOT, and hyaluronic acid injections are already making waves, in addition to the stem-cell therapies discussed previously, and we can expect them to be available cheaply and universally in the future. Similarly, it is important to consider cannabis, to stop demonizing this wonderful herb and realize how beneficial it can be.

The world of regenerative medicine has a lot of potential for growth. Be it through high-tech futuristic solutions such as 3-D bioprinting and stem cells or through ancient therapies such as cannabis, we are discovering and rediscovering ways of treating diseases that go beyond the symptom management approach of traditional allopathic medicine.

When considering such alternative medicine it is important to keep an open mind and to do enough research before trying it out. The mainstream medical community is conservative by nature and doesn't take kindly to new therapies but there is value in being careful when trying such alternate therapies.

REFERENCES FOR CHAPTER 15

American Chemical Society. "Exploring 3-D Printing to Make Organs for Transplants." *Science Daily,* July 30, 2014. www.sciencedaily.com/releases/2014/07/140730104140.htm (accessed May 6, 2017).

Boggs, Will. "3D 'Bioprinter' Produces Bone, Muscle, and Cartilage." *Reuters,* February 16, 2016. http://in.reuters.com/article/us-health-biotech-3d-printers-idINKCN0VO28X (accessed May 6, 2017).

Bushak, Lecia. "A Brief History of Medical Cannabis: From Ancient Anesthesia to the Modern Dispensary." *Medical Daily,* January 21, 2016. www.medicaldaily.com/brief-history-medical-cannabis-ancient-anesthesia-modern-dispensary-370344 (accessed May 6, 2017).

Calabria, Stephen. "Treating Cancer with Cannabis? Here Is What the Experts Say." *Green Flower,* March 3, 2016. http://greenflowermedia.com/article/treating-cancer-with-cannabis-2016-3/ (accessed May 6, 2017).

Deckoff-Jones, Jamie. "Hyperbaric Oxygen Therapy Is so Effective It Is a

Threat to Medicine, so FDA Moves to Restrict It." Healthimpactnews
.com, February 16, 2016. https://healthimpactnews.com/2013/hyperbaric
-oxygen-therapy-is-so-effective-it-is-a-threat-to-medicine-so-fda-moves-to
-restrict-it/ (accessed May 6, 2017).

EuroNews. "China Conducts First 3D Printed Vertebra Implant." January 9,
2014. www.euronews.com/2014/09/01/china-conducts-first-3d-printed
-vertebra-implant/ (accessed May 6, 2017).

Genece, Clifford. "Marijuana Legalization: 8 Ways CBD Can Change Your
Life." Honey Colony, July 6, 2016. www.honeycolony.com/article/10-ways
-cbd-marijuana-legalization-may-change-your-life/ (accessed May 6, 2017).

Greely, Henry T. "Putting Human Stem Cells in Animal Embryos? The NIH
Should Get on Board." *Los Angeles Times,* April 7, 2016. www.latimes
.com/opinion/op-ed/la-oe-0407-greely-human-animal-stem-cell-research
-20160407-story.html (accessed May 6, 2017).

HealthyCures.org. "5 Amazing Facts About Cannabis." December 29, 2015.
healthycures.org/5-amazing-facts-about-cannabis (accessed May 6, 2017).

HealthyCures.org. "9 Types of Cancer That Can Be Killed Cannabis (Here's
How)." September 11, 2015. http://healthycures.org/9-types-of-cancer-that
-can-be-killed-by-cannabis (accessed May 6, 2017).

Mercola, Joseph. "What Happens to Your Body When You Use Medical
Marijuana?" *Mercola,* February 7, 2016. http://articles.mercola.com/medical
-marijuana-uses.aspx (accessed May 6, 2017).

Moon, Mariella. "What You Need to Know about 3D Printed Organs."
Engadget, June 20, 2014. www.engadget.com/2014/06/20/3d-printed
-organ-explainer/ (accessed May 6, 2017).

Pfrommer, Rick. "Beginner's Guide to the Endocannabinoid System: The Reason
Our Bodies So Easily Process Cannabis." April 14, 2015. reset.me/story
/beginners-guide-to-the-endocannabinoid-system/ (accessed May 6, 2017).

Seshata. "Top 5 Benefits of Cannabis for Alzheimer's Disease." *Sensi Seeds,*
February 21, 2015. https://sensiseeds.com/en/blog/top-5-benefits-cannabis
-alzheimers-disease/ (accessed May 6, 2017).

PART 4

Take Charge of Your Life

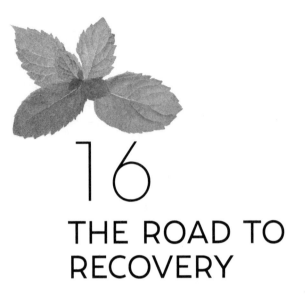

16

THE ROAD TO RECOVERY

The roots of all goodness lie in the soil of appreciation of goodness.

DALAI LAMA

Gratitude unlocks the fullness of life. It turns what we have into enough, and more. It turns denial into acceptance, chaos to order, confusion to clarity. It can turn a meal into a feast, a house into a home, a stranger into a friend. Gratitude makes sense of our past, brings peace for today and creates a vision for tomorrow.

MELODIE BEATTIE

Grace Bluerock served as a hospice nurse for many years. As she sat next to men and women who were dying, she couldn't help but listen to their final joys and regrets. It broke her heart to know that these people really could have made choices to live a happier and more contented life. As they lay there in their final days and hours, they spoke their regrets.

For some, they regretted not being kinder to the people they were supposed to have loved. For others, they regretted not spending quality time with their loved ones. If they had worked less and spent more time with their family, they would have been happier. Others regretted playing it safe and not pursuing their dreams in life. If they had only taken the time to be more carefree and taken a few more chances, they may have lived a happier life. The stories went on and on.

While Grace sat at their sides and listened to their last regrets, she knew that she wouldn't find herself regretting her choices when it was too late. She made the conscious decision to live her life to the fullest. She would show love to those that mattered most in her life. She would wake up being grateful for a new day.

The most important thing to take away from spending time with a hospice patient is that you need to live your life so that you die with no regrets. Be thankful for what you have and show your loved ones how much they really mean to you!

Many older people are isolated, lonely, and depressed. With more people living alone and longer, and many of us over-reliant on the internet for human interaction, loneliness is on the rise. Loneliness now affects 40 percent of the population. This phenomenon has some severe health consequences. Your interactions and attitude toward other people can have a big effect on your health. Being lonely increases the risk of everything from heart attacks to dementia, depression, and death. People who are satisfied with their social lives and connections not only sleep better but also age more slowly. Ameliorating loneliness is good for your health.

Loneliness can be caused by the death of a spouse, the children leaving, poverty, mobility and health issues, technology, geographical isolation, and having a lack of life goals. Many seniors cope with their loneliness by drinking and other activities that help fill the void. They also find that they get sick more often or find themselves overly concerned with health issues.

Loneliness now affects 40 percent of the population.

In this chapter, we will examine how loneliness can be ameliorated not only through increased social contact but also by certain emotional traits.

We will examine the role of gratitude, altruism, kindness, resiliency, a sense of purpose, laughter, volunteering, positive thinking, and spirituality. All of these factors can help alleviate the loneliness trend and help fill the void when life doesn't seem as fulfilling as you would like it to be.

WHY BE GRATEFUL?

Remember, if you are criticizing, you are not being grateful. If you are blaming, you are not being grateful. If you are complaining, you are not being grateful. If you are feeling tension, you are not being grateful. If you are rushing, you are not being grateful. If you are in a bad mood, you are not being grateful. Gratitude can transform your life. Are you allowing minor things to get in the way of your transformation and the life you deserve?

RHONDA BYRNE, *THE SECRET*

Everyone wants to have a happier and more fulfilling life. However, not many people realize that goal. The sad part about this is that they ultimately do this to themselves. How so? Attitude is one of the key elements in being happy and satisfied in your life. Those who are more grateful tend to be happier, experience less disease, and experience many more positive things in their lives.

Science has found that 50 percent of our ability to feel gratitude is genetic predisposition. That means that the other 50 percent is up to how we choose to live our lives and how we view what is going on around us. By engaging in activities that promote gratitude and surrounding ourselves with people who influence happiness in us, we are one step closer to making that 50 percent the best that it can possibly be. Just because you may suffer from genetic depression doesn't mean that you cannot be grateful. You just need to work with the factors in your life that you can control.

We hear about gratitude and being grateful all the time. What is the difference between gratitude and thankfulness? According to Dr. Mercola, "Gratitude is a thankful appreciation for what an individual receives, whether tangible or intangible. With gratitude, people acknowledge the goodness in their lives." Being thankful is just on the surface. Gratitude goes much deeper. You have the deep satisfaction of knowing that you are truly thankful for what you have.

> **Being thankful is just on the surface. Gratitude goes much deeper.**

Gratitude also has a lot to do with acceptance. Accepting what you have and being thankful for it is important for true gratitude. Acceptance does not mean resignation to your present situation and not trying to improve it. Acceptance means to be thankful for what you already have and then from this point of positivity to go forward and try to become better and get better things. When you pursue success from a place of gratitude you will be much happier with the results than if you were to pursue success from a place of anger or sadness about your current situation.

Gratitude brings positivity in your life. It keeps you happy, no matter what your situation is. And when you achieve success with gratitude, it is long lasting and you will never take it for granted.

Benefits of Gratitude

Gratitude practice isn't just about being happy. A grateful person can be healthier and live longer than someone who experiences negativity and depression. Studies have proven that those who show their gratitude more frequently have less chance of becoming ill and experiencing headaches, and instead live an overall happier life. So, what are some of the other benefits of showing gratitude on a regular basis?

Gratitude can:

- Help you cope with stress
- Allow you to show caring toward others
- Strengthen relationships
- Raise your self-esteem and self-image
- Help you sleep better
- Help alleviate health problems, mainly dealing with cardiovascular health

In one study, Professor Paul Mills studied a total of 186 men and women to see what the effects of gratitude were on their cardiovascular health. This group of people had already experienced problems with their cardiovascular health. Mills began by administering a survey on how grateful these people really were. He noticed that the more grateful they were, the fewer health problems they encountered. Going further, Mills did blood tests on those participating in the study and found that there was less inflammation in those who experienced more gratitude in their daily lives.

In another study, Mills had forty individuals who had cardiovascular health problems keep a gratitude journal for a month. At the end of the month, those who took part in the study were feeling better and experiencing fewer cardiovascular symptoms. Gratitude played a large part in improving existing health conditions!

People who are grateful for what they have are magnets for those who are seeking meaning and happiness in their own lives. Learning to live a life of gratitude can not only help you to be happier and healthier, it can also influence the moods of those around you.

When peeople are truly grateful for what they have in their lives, it shows. There is a deep sense of contentment in what they say or do. You can tell that a grateful person is a happy person. Since there are so many benefits to gratitude, why not find what you're grateful for and focus on these things rather than the frustrations of life? Let's look at some ways in which you can find what you're grateful for and recognize how these things impact your life.

FINDING GRATITUDE

Being grateful in some of life's circumstances may be incredibly difficult. Finding ways and things to be grateful for will help you to look at the small things in your life that are fulfilling and worth living for. Sometimes, it may take some effort to find things in your life that you can honestly say that you are grateful for. With some effort, you are able to grasp at a few good elements of your life. That's a start.

Planting and nurturing gratitude in your daily life will soon make it easier to find areas that you can honestly say you're grateful for. Find those few things that you can show gratitude for. Write them down. Some people even carry around a gratitude journal so that they can write down things for which they are grateful. When you recognize something that you can truly say you're grateful for, the other areas in your life to show gratitude for will become more apparent to you.

A good way to find things to be grateful for is to look at others less fortunate than yourself. There are billions of people in the world who have absolutely nothing. They live in areas torn apart by war or famine and just surviving is a struggle. Compared to these people, anyone who has a roof over his or her head, access to food, clean water, and loved ones around him or her, is incredibly lucky and should be grateful for all this. If you look hard enough you can always find a lot of things to be grateful for in your life.

Meditation

Sometimes, we may not realize that we are grateful for something at first. We really have to dig deep into our minds to bring to the surface the areas in our lives that we are grateful for. If you cannot quote everything that you're grateful for in one sentence, you're not the only one. Finding areas to be grateful for in your life may take some thought.

People have found that taking some quiet time and meditating on what they are grateful for has helped them bring feelings of deep gratitude to their consciousness.

Meditation helps to calm your chaotic mind so you can connect with yourself. We are so busy in our daily lives and there are so many things in the outside world demanding our attention that we forget to pay attention to ourselves. Meditation helps you to make time for yourself.

You don't even have to be into spirituality to meditate. Just take ten to fifteen minutes in the morning to sit in a quiet place and try to calm your mind by focusing on your breath. When a thought arises, as it surely will, just remind yourself to let it go. Slowly the superficial thoughts about work and what someone said about you and relationships and other issues will fade away and deeper thoughts will rise that will show you who you truly are and this can help you to find things that you can be grateful for.

Showing Gratitude

You may feel gratitude, but that really means nothing until you can begin to show gratitude in your daily life. Showing how you're grateful and practicing gratitude can help the feeling become a part of your daily life, not just something that you focus on and then go on with the way your life was before.

What are you grateful for? Try focusing your gratitude on things other than the material objects you possess. Think of relationships or experiences that you have had. Having a deeper sense of gratitude goes far beyond what we can possess. It really has to do with those we love and how we share our time with them. True gratitude takes the focus off ourselves and puts it on the way we experience the lives that we are given.

Start by showing gratitude to strangers for their service. Say *thank you* and *please* to everyone you interact with. A thank you can not only brighten up the day of a food server but it will also help you get in the habit of showing gratitude. If you can say thank you to strangers, you must also say it to your family when they do things for you. Once you get used to that, it is just one step more to start telling your family and loved ones how much they mean to you and how thankful you are for their presence in your life. It will improve your relationships and also help you feel more gratitude in your life, which will keep you healthy.

Gratitude Time

It may feel silly to you, but having a time where you point out what you're grateful for and why can significantly help you practice gratitude on a daily basis. Many people will take this gratitude time to reflect upon their lives and their circumstances in order to determine what they are grateful for and why. Those who make gratitude time a regular practice find that they are more genuine when they say that they really are thankful for what they have and for the people and the means that got them there.

Try taking some time in your day and set it as gratitude time. Sit and think about the things in your life that you are grateful to have. Think of the people and the relationships that make you who you are. By recognizing and pointing to the people and things that make you feel gratitude, you will feel a more positive attitude toward the negative aspects of life. For the most part, people really do not take the time to realize just how much they have. In our society we are told to focus on the things we want to get and not on the things we already have. Even when we get something we coveted for years, we quickly forget about it and move on to the next object. This isn't very healthy and leads to negativity and depression when you always focus on the things you don't have. More people would be happier and healthier if they would practice gratitude time.

HOW KINDNESS AND GRATITUDE WORK TOGETHER

The simplest acts of kindness are far more powerful than a thousand heads bowing in prayer.

MAHATMA GANDHI

Gratitude can be shown in many different ways. Showing gratitude generally allows you to display kindness to another person for whom you are grateful. By doing acts of kindness toward others, you are showing them that you are grateful for them and for what they represent in your life. Has someone ever shown you his or her gratitude by doing something kind for you?

Kindness and gratitude really go hand in hand. In order to show gratitude, you will have to be kind. You may feel grateful, but showing kindness is another facet to making gratitude affect your health in positive ways. Let's take a look at some ways in which you can show your gratitude through kindness and allow others to be grateful as well.

Practicing Acts of Kindness

My religion is very simple. My religion is kindness.

DALAI LAMA

One of the basic points is kindness. With kindness, with love and compassion, with this feeling that is the essence of brotherhood, sisterhood, one will have inner peace. This compassionate feeling is the basis of inner peace.

DALAI LAMA

Giving as well as receiving kindness builds the full benefits of how gratitude can affect your happiness and your health. Try showing people that you're grateful for something that they have done. It doesn't have to be a big gesture, but it can be something small that shows them that you notice them and all that they do.

When trying to show your gratitude, try expressing it through acts of kindness. There are many ways in which you can show that you're grateful for what people do for you. You can:

- Leave a thank you note
- Give them a small gift
- Tell them that you really appreciate their work, no matter how small the task was
- Bring up their achievements in front of others to show how great you thought they were
- Show kindness in other ways, like by doing something you know they will appreciate, going out of your way to accommodate them, and showing through your actions that you care for them and consider their feelings in your decision-making process

Simple acts of kindness will not only make someone else feel better, but they will also help you feel better. There is something about cheering people up and making their day that will lift your own spirits and help you to feel happier and more joyful.

Think of ways that you can practice kindness toward those you care about. You can even show kindness to strangers. Just knowing that you notice and appreciate people and their actions can really boost their spirits and yours as well!

Benefits of Kindness

Whether one believes in a religion or not, and whether one believes in rebirth or not, there isn't anyone who doesn't appreciate kindness and compassion.

DALAI LAMA

Just like there are benefits to gratitude, there are also some nice benefits to being kind. People may see those who are kind as being weak and easily taken advantage of, but little do they realize, the people who show kindness on a regular basis are actually healthier and happier than those who are selfish and negative! So, what are some benefits to showing kindness?

Showing kindness can:

- Make you happier
- Help build a healthier heart
- Decrease aging
- Build stronger relationships
- Produce kindness in others
- Make you live longer
- Have positive effects on your brain

Just like showing gratitude, showing kindness can also have great health benefits. It makes for a happier and positive lifestyle. Who wouldn't want to be healthier and happier? Take some time to show some kindness to those around you!

Kindness and gratitude really work hand in hand. Those you are kind to also know that you are grateful that they are a part of your life and that they matter to you. Even if they are strangers to you, they will appreciate kindness. Don't discount acts of kindness. They may be just what someone needs to get out of a deep depression or look at the bright side of a crummy day!

> *When we feel love and kindness toward others, it not only makes others feel loved and cared for, but it helps us also to develop inner happiness and peace.*
>
> Dalai Lama

BEING CONTENT WITH YOUR LIFE AND HAVING PURPOSE

Along with being grateful for your life and what you have, it is incredibly important that you are content with what you have. You can say that you're content and grateful, but you may not necessarily experience both feelings. A true contentment with your life will lead to gratitude. There are many people out there who say that they are grateful, but they really lack contentment with their lives. This can inhibit the benefits of gratitude. So, how can you know whether or not you're content with your life?

Contentment comes through acceptance. If you are not financially well off and want to earn more, then you won't be content with your life. But this will drive negativity in your life and stop you from being grateful. Accepting what you already have is completely possible while also wanting more. You can want more in one area of your life while simultaneously being content with your life in general. This is a much more positive way of approaching life and will keep you healthy and happy.

Finding Your Purpose

You will find people who really know that they are grateful for their lives. When asked why they know this, they will respond with the fact that they know their purpose in life and are living that purpose. It may be difficult for you to pinpoint your own purpose in life. Everyone has a purpose for being here. If you find that you cannot think of your purpose at this very moment, place your hand over your heart. Feel your heart beating? That is enough purpose to get you through a day!

Take a look around you. Think about your life. There are many purposes you serve. You may be someone's mother. You may be someone's best friend who helps him or her through a tough day. There are so many purposes you serve just by being you. Find these little things and let them become your source of gratitude! If you have trouble finding your purpose, try meditating on ways you fit into the world. If you are spiritual, pray about where God wants you to serve. Really dig deep and think about how the world is a better place because of you. This might be the purpose that you serve in life.

If you can't find a purpose, give yourself one. Having a self-appointed purpose can be just as powerful as finding a purpose through a life-changing epiphany. Once you start following this purpose, maybe it will become your real purpose. If not, it will help you to get closer to your real purpose.

Once you have found your purpose, live for it. Let your purpose be a positive light for others to follow. Finding your purpose will allow you to feel more content, and it will also allow you to show your light to the world.

Having a Purpose Helps You Live Longer

Just like gratitude and kindness, purpose will also add years to your life. Those who know their purpose and live for these purposes have a deeper sense of contentment, which eases stress and depression. Ultimately, having lower levels of stress and easing depression can have dramatic effects on your overall health! Those who have a strong purpose in their lives actually live longer than those just trying to make it through life!

Make your life one without regrets.

Take time to be grateful, be kinder to others, and find your purpose in life. Make your life one without regrets. Just like the hospice nurse in the opening of this chapter, find a reason to live your life to the fullest and put your efforts where they truly matter. The decision is yours. Do it today. Don't wait until it's too late to be grateful for your life!

POINTS TO REMEMBER

Gratitude can be shown in many different ways. Finding and showing your gratitude can help you live a longer and more contented life. People who show gratitude are healthier and happier than those who feel negativity on a regular basis. Take time to not only realize what you're grateful for, but also show your gratitude and appreciation to others.

Acts of kindness are a wonderful way to show your true gratitude to others. It will help you feel happier and make those around you feel happier as well. Gratitude is a conscious choice. Who doesn't want to be healthier and happier? Taking the time to express gratitude will help you to feel happier, which in turn will help your overall health.

Knowing your purpose in life is another way in which you can find true contentment, which leads to gratitude. Do you struggle with finding contentment and gratitude in your daily life? It might be time to examine your life and find what you're here for. Take some time and find your purpose in life. Make each day a way to live out your purpose.

Gratitude, kindness, and purpose all lead to a longer and happier life. Learning to find these elements in your life will help you to become more positive and enjoy your life more.

I encourage you to take the time to really meditate and find the things that you are grateful for in life. Take these things and place your efforts into helping them flourish. The more content and grateful you are, the more likely you are to live a happier and healthier life. Don't wait until it's too late. Don't allow yourself to slip away from this life with regrets. Make conscious changes to your mind and lifestyle to help you enjoy your life more fully today!

REFERENCES FOR CHAPTER 16

Association for Psychological Science. "Having a Sense of Purpose May Add Years to Your Life." *Science Daily,* May 12, 2014. www.sciencedaily.com/releases/2014/05/140512124308.htm (accessed May 6, 2007).

Bluerock, Grace. "The 9 Most Common Regrets People Have at the End of Life." *MindBodyGreen,* January 2, 2016. www.mindbodygreen.com/0-23024/the-9-most-common-regrets-people-have-at-the-end-of-life.html (accessed May 6, 2007).

Bourne, Sue. "10 Reasons People Are Lonely? It's More Complicated Than That." *Guardian,* January 4, 2016. www.theguardian.com/commentisfree/2016/jan/04/10-reasons-people-lonely-the-age-of-loneliness (accessed May 6, 2007).

Castillo, Stephanie. "The Science of Gratitude: It Really Is the Little Things." *Medical Daily,* November 13, 2014. www.medicaldaily.com/science-gratitude-it-really-little-things-310468 (accessed May 6, 2007).

Field, Peter. "5 Researched-Based Reasons to Be Kind." *HuffPost,* April 20, 2015. www.huffingtonpost.com/peter-field/kindness-research_b_7054652.html (accessed May 6, 2007).

Froelich, Amanda. "Really, Science Proves Being Grateful Improves Your Health." *True Activist,* February 21, 2015. www.trueactivist.com/really-science-proves-being-grateful-improves-your-health/ (accessed May 6, 2007).

Haas, Michaela. "Want to Be Happy? Practice Gratitude. Here's How." *MindBodyGreen,* November 26, 2015. www.mindbodygreen.com/0-22370 /want-to-be-happy-practice-gratitude-heres-how.html (accessed May 6, 2007).

Hamilton, D. R. "5 Beneficial Side Effects of Kindness." *HuffPost,* June 2, 2011. www.huffingtonpost.com/david-r-hamilton-phd/kindness-benefits_b_869537 .html (accessed May 6, 2007).

Hill, P. L. "Purpose in Life Adds Years to Life." WorldHealth.net, June 20, 2014. www.worldhealth.net/news/purpose-life-adds-years-life/ (accessed May 6, 2007).

Mercola, Joseph. "Kindness: Just the Opposite of Killing Us; It Makes Us Stronger." *Mercola,* July 4, 2013. http://articles.mercola.com/sites/articles /archive/2013/07/04/kindness.aspx (accessed May 6, 2007).

———. "The Many Benefits of Expressing and Receiving Gratitude." *Mercola,* November 26, 2015. http://articles.mercola.com/sites/articles /archive/2015/11/26/expressing-gratitude.aspx (accessed May 6, 2007).

Murray, Michael T. "You've Heard Gratitude Is Good for You. Here's What Science Says." *MindBodyGreen,* March 29, 2015. www.mindbodygreen .com/0-18054/youve-heard-gratitude-is-good-for-you-heres-what-science -says.html (accessed May 6, 2007).

Neighmond, Patti. "Gratitude Is Good for the Soul and Helps the Heart, Too." November 23, 2015. www.mprnews.org/story/npr/456656055 (accessed May 6, 2007).

17
REGENERATIVE RECIPES

One cannot think well, love well, sleep well, if one has not dined well.

VIRGINIA WOOLF

Most of us not only want to look as young as possible, but also feel young. We discussed many of the regenerative strategies in this book. At the top of the list of things to do to stay young is maintaining a healthy and well-balanced diet. This chapter was written with the idea of presenting a selection of tempting natural food recipes for people who are concerned about their health and are beginning to make a natural transition to a more healthy way of eating.

**Food is not just supposed to be healthy,
but also delicious.**

When I moved from New York to California, I began teaching classes in cooking, using the abundance of fresh natural fruits and vegetables available in Southern California. My intention was not so much to teach people how to cook (as I believe cooking is an intuitive art), but to share recipes in order to inspire students to create their own original recipes using locally grown natural ingredients.

It is said there is a language of flowers, but there is also a language of foods. The recipes included in this chapter represent the best from my classes, adaptations of ethnic foods from my childhood, and creative recipes I've presented to friends within my own home. I know you will enjoy them. I would like to suggest that after the initial testing of a new recipe, you trust your intuition and allow yourself greater freedom in its preparation.

My cooking classes evolved out of my own transition to eating a more natural and healthy diet. I stopped eating refined and processed foods, white flour, sugar, and meat, and began to substitute these with healthier foods. It was then that I discovered the exciting challenge of taking the traditional recipes of my childhood and adapting them to fit my tastes. Mealtime became not only more healthful, but also a delicious adventure. I also discovered natural foods to be so versatile in taste and texture that I happily used them in place of processed ingredients in my cooking. I invite you to start by trying these recipes, and then begin to create your own.

While I was teaching cooking at the Los Angeles City Colleges for nine years, I found that people were very aware of what foods constituted good nutrition and what foods to eliminate. However, what they really wanted were some guidelines. They were not interested in spending long hours cooking or making meals that required many ingredients or many steps. Over the years, I have developed tried-and-true recipes that not only are easy to prepare, but are also delicious and healthy. Many years after I gave up teaching to spend more time in private practice, I often encountered former students who would tell me that they were still making the dishes they learned in my cooking classes. In this chapter, I enclose some of the most popular recipes for breakfast, lunch, dinner, and dessert. All of these dishes use many of the traditional foods of our ancestors.

The premise of this chapter is that food is not just supposed to be healthy for us, but also delicious. I hope these recipes will inspire you to create some of your own.

BREAKFAST RECIPES

As it is commonly quoted, "Breakfast is the most important meal of the day." In a sense, this is absolutely true. Since food is fuel for the body, it's important to fuel your body when you first wake up in the morning. Having a solid breakfast is important for your health and energy levels throughout the day. It can also be one of the most enjoyable meals of the day. Learning to cook with healthy ingredients will help you to enjoy your food while easing inflammation. Also, eating better now could mean a longer and healthier life!

Let's take a look at some of my favorite breakfast recipes that include healthy and flavorful food. Once you have tried these, you probably won't go back to the processed and sugary breakfast foods that are so popular!

🖋 BREAKFAST SHAKE

Ingredients

16 oz. of liquid. This can be straight water or a combination of water and soy or coconut milk.

2 TBSP of ground flax meal

2 TBSP chia seeds

½ TBSP of unsweetened cocoa powder

½ cup of fresh blueberries

1 cup of organic greens such as kale, spinach, and chard

3 ice cubes

Stevia sweetener to taste

Directions for Preparation

Combine ingredients in a blender and blend on high speed until they are mixed to satisfaction.

🖋 EGG MUFFINS

With this recipe, you have the freedom of deciding what meat, vegetables, and cheeses you put into it. Find a combo that you enjoy and let this become a breakfast go to!

Ingredients

1 chopped onion

1 chopped tomato

Cheese of choice

Green chili if desired

6 eggs, beaten with 2 TBSP of milk and black pepper to taste

You can add lean meat or other vegetables as desired!

Directions for Preparation

Start by preheating your oven to 400°F. Grease your muffin pan. Take your meat and vegetable mixture and cheese, and put in the muffin molds. Pour your egg mixture over the vegetables. Bake for 20–25 minutes. Make sure that the edges are brown and set before removing from the oven. Allow to cool for about 10 minutes. Remove from pan and either enjoy or freeze for later!

🌿 BREAKFAST BARS

If you're looking for a breakfast you can grab on the go, look no further! These are both superhealthy and superconvenient!

Ingredients

8 dates, chopped

¼ cup raw sunflower seeds

¼ cup raw almonds

¼ cup shredded coconut

1–2 TBSP coconut oil, softened

Small amount of salt

1 TBSP chia seeds

2 TBSP cacao nibs

Optional: coconut butter, softened

Directions for Preparation

Combine dates, sunflower seeds, almonds, shredded coconut, coconut oil, and salt in food processor until a suitable batter forms. Start the food processor with 1 TBSP coconut oil and add more if blending is difficult. After well combined, transfer to bowl and stir chia seeds and cacao nibs into batter.

Use hands to form batter into rectangular shape on baking sheet. Take formed batter and place in freezer for about 10 minutes to harden.

Remove and slice into bars. Drizzle or spread coconut butter on top. Store in refrigerator until ready to serve.

*   OATMEAL BREAKFAST CAKE

Let's face it: there are two types of breakfast people. Some like the eggs and meat, while others like the sweet side of the meal. This recipe is perfect for those who enjoy a sweet and healthy breakfast!

Ingredients

½ cup oats

I cup water

3 TBSP coconut oil

¼ cup unsweetened applesauce

I egg

2 egg whites

2 TSP vanilla extract

¼ cup walnuts, finely chopped

¼ cup raisins, finely chopped

⅔ cup sugar or equivalent of stevia

I cup whole wheat flour

2 TBSP protein powder

2 TSP cinnamon

½ TSP allspice

½ TSP salt

I TSP baking soda

Directions for Preparation

Preheat oven to 350°F. Spray an 8 x 8 baking pan with nonstick cooking spray. Set aside. Prepare the oatmeal as usual in a large bowl, using I cup of water. Stir in the coconut oil, applesauce, egg, egg whites, vanilla, walnuts, raisins, and sugar or stevia.

In a separate bowl, mix together protein powder, flour, cinnamon, allspice, salt, and baking soda.

Combine all the dry ingredients with wet ingredients and stir until well mixed.

Pour mixture into baking pan. Bake for 25–30 minutes or until knife inserted in center comes out clean.

Remove from oven and let cool. Cut into 6 squares and serve.

LUNCH RECIPES

By the time we reach lunch hour, we are usually famished. It may seem easier to hit the local burger joint and order the greasy, tasty fare, but it really isn't healthy and your body will tell you about it later. There are ways to eat a healthy and fulfilling lunch without the temptation of hitting the drive-thru. Preparing your lunches at home can really help you to take your healthy diet along with you. Just because you have a short amount of time to eat lunch does not mean that it has to lack in nutrition!

In this section, I am going to share some of my favorite lunch recipes. These not only taste great, but they will also give your body the nutrients it needs to fuel the rest of your day. Try a few of these tasty recipes and see and feel the benefits!

🌿 ZUCCHINI PANCAKES

These tasteful and easy pancakes can be served as a side or as the main meal. They are filling and will complement your lunch nicely!

Ingredients
2 TBSP olive oil
2 medium zucchinis, grated and well drained
1 carrot, grated
½ cup chopped green onions
1–2 eggs or egg whites, beaten
½ cup whole wheat pastry flour
Oregano, sweet basil, garlic powder, and tamari to taste

Directions for Preparation
Sauté carrot and zucchini in the olive oil until slightly limp. Make sure they are still bright in color. Mix zucchini and carrot with onion, eggs, flour, and herbs. Season with tamari to taste. Adjust seasonings to your liking.

Drop by tablespoon onto oiled, hot skillet. Pan fry until brown on both sides. You can serve these either hot or cold.

🖋 LEMON TAHINI DRESSING

This dressing makes a great addition to your leafy greens! It's light in flavor and easy to prepare!

Ingredients

2 cups olive oil

¼ cup bell pepper, chopped

1 stalk celery, chopped

1 clove of garlic

1 cup plus 1 TBSP lemon juice

½ TBSP or less tamari

½ cup tahini (raw)

¼ onion, chopped

Directions for Preparation

In food processor, blend vegetables until smooth. Add liquid ingredients and blend until creamy. Store in refrigerator.

🖋 TOFU BROWN RICE BURGERS

If you're in the mood for a good burger, give these a try! They taste great and are made with healthy ingredients.

Ingredients

1 lb. tofu, crumbled

2 cups cooked brown rice

2 cloves garlic, diced

Olive oil

1 large onion, chopped finely

1 carrot, grated

1–2 eggs (as binder)

Tamari (to taste)

½ cup whole wheat flour or wheat germ (as binder)

Directions for Preparation

Start by mashing your tofu in a bowl. Add cooked rice. Sauté garlic in the olive oil, adding onions and then carrots and cook until tender.

Mix your cooked vegetables with the tofu and rice. Beat your egg and add it to the tofu mixture. Use tamari to season to taste. Mix all together. If the mixture is too loose, add some wheat germ to bind it.

Form the mixture into patties and bake on oiled cookie sheet at 300°F until brown. These taste great served with the lemon tahini dressing!

🖋 CLASSIC FETA CHEESE SALAD

This is another light lunch salad that has a great Mediterranean feel to it. Using these fresh ingredients, you can enjoy a tasty and fresh lunch salad!

Ingredients

4 cucumbers
4 large tomatoes
1 medium red onion, diced small
2 TSP fresh parsley, chopped
Handful of black Israeli-style olives
Feta cheese, cubed

Ingredients for Dressing

2–3 TBSP olive oil
Juice of ½ lemon
1 TSP sea salt

Directions for Preparation

Start by cutting cucumbers and tomatoes into small cubes. Add diced red onion, parsley, olives, and feta cheese and mix all together gently. Cover with the dressing.

For the Israeli twist, you can add 2 TSP of chopped fresh mint and 1 TSP of zander.

🍃 TABOOLI

This recipe makes a great lunchtime oatmeal. Using anti-inflammatory ingredients, you can make a filling and healthy meal that you can enjoy on the go!

Ingredients

1 cup cracked wheat

2 cups water

⅓ cup parsley, minced

½ cup fresh mint leaves

½ cup green onions, finely chopped

5–6 TBSP olive oil

2–4 TBSP lemon juice

1 TSP salt

1 TSP allspice, or to taste

Tomatoes and red peppers for garnish

Directions for Preparation

Pour boiling water over wheat and cover tightly. Let sit 20 minutes until tender. Drain off any extra water. Add parsley, mint, and onion and toss to mix. Combine oil, lemon juice, salt, and allspice to taste. Add to wheat mixture. Chill. Serve with garnishments to add color.

🍃 PIAS DE AVAS

This bean salad can be served as a side or as the main dish.

Ingredients

1 cup small white beans

1 cup green onions, finely chopped

1 cup parsley, finely chopped

2 TBSP olive oil

3 TBSP cider vinegar

Salt to taste

Directions for Preparation

Soak beans overnight. Cook by boiling until tender. Drain well. Add onions, parsley, oil, and vinegar. Season to taste. Serve cold. This dish has improved flavor if marinated for a few hours.

🌿 SIMPLE CURRIED CHICKPEA SALAD

This salad can be served in many ways. From putting it on bread to eating it on crackers, this is sure to be a family favorite!

Ingredients

1 cup dried chickpeas, soaked then cooked until very tender, or two 15-oz. cans chickpeas, drained and rinsed

3 celery ribs, diced small

1 large organic Granny Smith apple, peeled and diced small

½ cup toasted chopped pecans

½ cup currants or raisins

⅓ cup vegan mayonnaise

1 TBSP curry powder

2 whole scallions, green parts thinly sliced and white parts minced

1 large garlic clove, minced

Sea salt and freshly ground black pepper to taste

Directions for Preparation

To start, place half of the chickpeas in a food processor and pulse them once or twice to chop them up a bit. This can also be done in a bowl with a potato masher. Place the chickpeas and the rest of the salad ingredients in a large bowl and mix them with a rubber spatula until well combined. Season the salad with salt and pepper; then cover and refrigerate it for 30 minutes before serving.

DINNER RECIPES

Dinner is a time for you and your family to sit together and share stories about your day. If you are traditional, this takes place around a table with food being passed around. The food always tastes great and the company makes it even better. This is one of the memories that frequently is related when we talk to centenarians about their diets. What kind of food was passed around the table in your home when you were growing up?

Having a family dinner with warm food and conversation will make eating not only tasty, but enjoyable. In this section, I'm going to share with you some of my favorite dinner recipes that will give you the taste and the health benefits, so you too can share your dinnertime memories when you're a centenarian. Find the recipes that you enjoy from this chapter and make them your new family favorites!

🌿 RATATOUILLE

This recipe gives you a marinara sauce that can be used with your favorite dishes. The fresh ingredients and the seasonings will have you begging for more!

Ingredients

2 TBSP olive oil

2 large cloves of garlic, diced

1 large onion, diced

3 medium zucchini, thickly sliced

½ medium eggplant cut into ½-inch cubes

One red or green bell pepper, seeded and diced

2 cups spaghetti sauce

Seasonings to taste: sweet basil, oregano, and tamari

Directions for Preparation

Sauté garlic in oil. Add onion and continue to sauté until golden brown. Toss in zucchini, eggplant, and pepper. Continue cooking until vegetables are slightly limp. Add spaghetti sauce and season to taste with herbs.

🌿 STUFFED EGGPLANT

Eggplant is one of the best vegetables to eat when looking for healthy food. It's rich in antioxidants and can be served in a variety of ways. This recipe will allow you to serve it as a main dish.

Ingredients

4 small eggplants, cut lengthwise

Oil for sautéing

1 clove garlic, chopped

1 bunch scallions

½ lb. tofu drained and cubed

2 cups cooked rice

Tamari soy sauce

Garlic powder to taste

Directions for Preparation

Cut washed eggplants in half lengthwise and steam in about 1 inch of water until pulp is tender and color changes. With a teaspoon, gently scoop out the pulp, leaving ¼-inch border of skin. Chop pulp.

In another pan, in 2 tablespoons of oil, sauté scallions and tofu. Add rice and continue to sauté until brown. Add 2 capfuls of tamari and add garlic powder to taste. Combine chopped eggplant pulp and rice mixture and spoon into the hollowed eggplants. Bake at 350°F for 30 minutes or until golden brown.

✿ QUINOA FRIED RICE

Ingredients

1 box white quinoa (about 2 cups)
1 box frozen peas
1 red pepper, chopped
1 white onion, chopped
1 8-oz. can baby corn
2 orange carrots, chopped
1 8-oz. can sliced water chestnuts
1 TBSP regular sesame oil (or olive oil)
3 eggs, certified humane or pasture raised
Dash of sea salt
4 TBSP tamari
3 TBSP toasted sesame oil
2 scallions, chopped
2 TBSP white sesame seeds

Directions for Preparation

Rinse quinoa and cook according to package directions. Thaw peas by running them under cold water in a colander. In a large pan, sauté peas and chopped veggies with 2 tablespoons of sesame oil. Once veggies are fully cooked, add cooked quinoa and stir together.

Make a little hole in the center of the veggie-quinoa mixture and crack eggs. Scramble the egg with sea salt in the center of the pan. Let everything cook and then stir it around with the quinoa mixture so everything is mixed together.

Sprinkle tamari, toasted sesame oil, scallions, and sesame seeds on top. Serve with chopsticks and enjoy!

🖊 BAKED POTATO SOUP

Ingredients

I large russet potato, baked and cooled

I cup chicken or vegetable broth

½ cup onion, minced

¼ cup onion tops, chopped

¼ cup butter

I cup sour cream

7 cups of your favorite milk

Directions for Preparation

Remove potato skin, including about ¼ inch of the potato and discard the remainder of the potato. Blend the potato skins with the chicken broth in blender or food processor. Combine the onion, butter, and a little chicken broth and sauté until onions are tender. Add the onion mixture to the blended potato mixture with the milk and blend until smooth. Pour the soup into a large pot and heat until very hot. It's now ready to serve! Top with sour cream and enjoy!

🖊 SPINACH AND GOAT CHEESE FRITTATA

Ingredients

3 TBSP olive oil

½ medium onion, thinly sliced

Small amounts of kosher salt and black pepper

5 ounces of baby spinach

10 large eggs, beaten

4 ounces goat cheese, crumbled

I TBSP white onion vinegar

Bread for serving

Directions for Preparation

Preheat the oven to 400°F. While oven is heating, heat I tablespoon of oil in a medium skillet over medium to high heat. Add the onion and ½ TSP each of salt and pepper. Let it cook, stirring occasionally. Wait for it to become golden brown, about 3 to 4 minutes.

Add the spinach to the skillet and cook, tossing the mixture until the spinach is wilted. Add the eggs and sprinkle with goat cheese. Continue to cook until the mixture begins to set around the edges. Put the skillet in the oven and bake for about 10–12 minutes.

Divide evenly and place on plates. Drizzle with vinegar and the remaining oil. Season to taste with salt and pepper. Serve with bread.

DESSERT RECIPES

Everyone loves dessert, right? Even if you are following a whole-foods diet, there can still be dessert involved. In this section, I am going to share some of my favorite dessert recipes for you to enjoy. What a great way to end your day! Enjoy a wonderful, healthy, and tasty dessert!

🌿 FRUIT SORBET
Just like ice cream, without the sugar! Fruit sorbet is a creamy treat and can be healthy as well!

Ingredients
Very ripe bananas
Pineapple

Toppings
Organic peanut butter cups
Organic chocolate chips
Pecans
Macadamia nuts
Pineapple puree

Directions for Preparation
Banana sorbet: Peel bananas and put in freezer. Once frozen, place bananas in juicer or blender and blend them. Spoon into dishes and add your toppings!

Pineapple sorbet: Peel pineapple and chop into chunks. Place in freezer. Once frozen, put in juicer or blender and blend. Put into serving dishes and add your favorite toppings! Enjoy!

🖋 LEMON COCONUT PUDDING

Ingredients

2 cups young coconut

I TSP vanilla

I ½ TBSP lemon juice

½ TSP honey, to balance

I cup water, in increments

½ TSP lemon extract

½ TSP almond extract

2 drops stevia

I pinch sea salt

I cup ice cubes

Directions for Preparation

In a high-speed blender, blend all ingredients except ice, until smooth. Taste and adjust the sweetness, if necessary. Add the ice and blend again until cool and creamy. Serve in small dishes and garnish with lemon zest.

🖋 EASY PEANUT BUTTER CHOCOLATE CHIP BALLS

Ingredients

½ cup peanut butter

½ TBSP sugarless Dutch chocolate or cocoa powder

3 TBSP dark chocolate chips

½ cup unsweetened shredded coconut

Directions for Preparation

Combine peanut butter, cocoa powder, and chocolate chips until well blended. Form the mixture into small balls. Roll in shredded coconut. Refrigerate, serve chilled.

🖋 CHOCOLATE PEANUT BUTTER SPREAD

Ingredients

½ cup peanut butter

½ TBSP dark cocoa powder (preferably unsweetened)

Directions for Preparation

Blend or mix thoroughly. Spread on crackers, pancakes, or put in oatmeal.

🖋 PEANUT BUTTER AND MILLET GRANOLA BARS

Ingredients

I ½ cup puffed millet or brown rice cereal

¼ TSP cinnamon

I cup old-fashioned oats

¼ cup dried currants or raisins

¼ cup almonds or cashews, chopped

⅓ cup peanut butter, melted

⅓ cup brown rice syrup

1 TSP vanilla

Directions for Preparation

Preheat oven to 325°F. Make a sling with parchment paper and line an 8 x 8 pan with it. Then spray bottom and sides of pan with nonstick spray.

In a large bowl, stir together millet, oats, cinnamon, currants, and nuts.

In a small bowl, stir together brown rice syrup and peanut butter. Microwave the mixture for 10 seconds, stir, and then microwave for another 10 seconds. Stir in vanilla and pour over dry ingredients.

Mix thoroughly so all ingredients are coated. I use my hands to help this process. Press firmly into pan using the back of a spatula. (You want to make sure you pack them firmly so they stay together when finished.)

Bake for 6 minutes. Remove from oven, press down on top once more with spatula and set pan on wire rack to cool completely. Remove from pan and cut into even bars.

✐ HEALTHY GRANOLA BARS

Ingredients

1 cup packed dates, pitted

1 ¼ cup honey (may substitute maple syrup or agave)

¼ cup creamy salted natural peanut butter or almond butter

1 cup roasted unsalted almonds, loosely chopped

1 ½ cups rolled oats

Optional additions: chocolate chips, dried fruit, nuts, banana chips, vanilla.

Directions for Preparation

Process dates in a food processor until small bits remain. It should form a doughlike consistency.

Place oats, almonds, and dates in a bowl and set aside. Warm honey and peanut butter in a small saucepan over low heat.

Stir and pour over oat mixture and then mix, breaking up the dates to disperse throughout. Once thoroughly mixed, transfer to an 8 x 8 dish or other small pan lined with plastic wrap or parchment paper so they lift out easily.

Press down until uniformly flattened. Cover with parchment or plastic wrap, and let set in fridge or freezer for 15–20 minutes to harden.

Remove from pan and cut into even bars. Store in an airtight container for up to a week.

🖋 APPLE CRISP

Ingredients

4 apples

I cup raisins

I cup chopped walnuts

2 cups granola

I TBSP cinnamon

Juice of ½ lemon

Directions for Preparation

Preheat the oven to 350°F. Peel and thinly slice apples with knife or hand grater. Plump raisins by soaking them in a small amount of hot water. Sprinkle apples with cinnamon, nuts, and lemon juice. Combine with raisins. Put in an 8 x 8 sprayed casserole dish. Top with granola and cover. Bake until apples are soft. This will take about 20 minutes. Uncover and bake for another 10 minutes.

🖋 RICE PUDDING

Ingredients

I lb. tofu, drained

1–2 eggs

½ cup maple syrup

2 lemons

I TBSP vanilla

I cup cooked brown rice

I cup unsweetened, shredded coconut

½ cup raisins

Directions for Preparation

Preheat the oven to 350°F.

In a blender combine tofu, eggs, maple syrup, lemon juice and pulp, and vanilla. Blend until smooth.

In a large bowl combine brown rice, coconut, and raisins. Combine with blended mixture. Put into baking pan and bake for about 45 minutes to an hour. Serve cold.

POINTS TO REMEMBER

Just because food is healthy doesn't mean that it can't taste good! I encourage you to put my recipes to the test and see if you can find some new favorites. I have used these recipes in numerous cooking classes and I still prepare them for myself to this day. My students have all given me great feedback on these select recipes as well. Once you have gotten the hang of preparing food using healthy and fresh ingredients, I encourage you to make up your own recipes and make your own family favorites!

REFERENCES FOR CHAPTER 17

Cooking Israel. "Classic Israeli Salad." http://israelforever.org/israel/cooking/Israeli_Salad/ (accessed May 6, 2017).

Evans, Pete. "Lemon Coconut Pudding Recipe." *Mercola Recipes,* January 6, 2017. http://recipes.mercola.com/lemon-coconut-pudding-recipe.aspx (accessed May 6, 2017).

Falotico, Samantha. "Gluten Free Peanut Butter & Millet Granola Bars." *Lifestyle,* January 27, 2015. www.aol.com/article/2015/01/27/gluten-free-peanut-butter-and-millet-granola-bars/21135468/ (accessed May 6, 2017).

Frahn, Allison. "Oatmeal Breakfast Cake." *Fitness Rx,* January 29, 2015. www.fitnessrxwomen.com/nutrition/recipes/allis-slim-pickins/oatmeal-breakfast-cake/ (accessed May 6, 2017).

Keating, Lauren. "Quinoa Fried Rice: A Great Way to Use Leftover Ham." *Healthy Delicious,* December 2008. www.healthy-delicious.com/quinoa-fried-rice-recipe/ (accessed May 6, 2017).

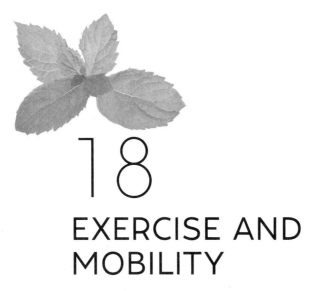

18

EXERCISE AND MOBILITY

If I'd known I was going to live this long, I'd have taken better care of myself.

EUBIE BLAKE

Those who do not find time for exercise will have to find time for illness.

EDWARD STANLEY

Regular exercise in later life can dramatically boost the chance of healthy aging, even for those who do not take up various physical activities until after they retire in their sixties. Statistics have shown that sustained and frequent physical activity raises the likelihood of people aging healthier than those who were physically inactive.

Staying physically fit not only lowers the risk of developing major diseases or disabilities, but also promotes positive mental health, prevents falling, and decreases the risk of dementia. Many older people do exercise regularly by walking, playing tennis, bowling, dancing, swimming, and in many other forms. All of these exercises are good and have many benefits.

However, there is a group of exercises that are gaining more popularity among active retirees because of their ability to improve balance and coordination, bring more flexibility and energy, and help increase the body's ability to heal.

In this chapter, we will examine yoga, t'ai chi, and qigong. These exercises have the power to increase energy, help us to feel calm, and invigorate us. These healing practices have been used for thousands of years, but it is only recently that scientists have begun to examine their effects on our brains and bodies.

When Elizabeth sat down in my office in Santa Barbara, I immediately noticed that she was not only overweight, but out of shape and not fit at all. Like many women in their sixties, she was not acculturated to exercise. Now in her late sixties, she was beginning to experience the effects of a sedentary lifestyle.

She complained of low energy, depression, difficulty losing weight, and "feeling old." And she looked a lot older than many of her contemporaries with her stooped posture and bulging belly. I asked what kind of exercise she did on a regular basis (already knowing the answer) and she said, "none" because she worked as a real estate agent, and her schedule was erratic. Many times when she wanted to go for a walk, it was already dark.

I suggested purchasing a treadmill. In this way, she could exercise at her convenience instead of worrying about getting to the gym or exercising when it was dark. She said she didn't have any room in her house for a treadmill. I suggested putting it in the garage.

When she came in for her follow-up visit a month later, she was smiling and said, "Thank you for suggesting the treadmill! It's the best thing ever. I walk before I go to work in the morning, while watching television, and even use it in the evening to unwind after a stressful day. I now have more energy and even lost five pounds!"

Take care of your body. It's the only place you have to live.

JIM ROHN

THE BENEFITS OF REGULAR EXERCISE FOR THOSE OVER THE AGE OF SIXTY

Sadly enough, many older people believe that their choices in early life dictate where they are right now. There is no use in changing their lifestyles because they are going to die soon anyway, right? Wrong! Even those who have made poor choices earlier in life can benefit by having a regular exercise routine.

Having a regular physical exercise routine for adults over sixty has proven to have incredible effects. Even if someone has had little to no physical activity prior to age sixty, studies have proven that those who take up a regular exercise routine in this older age will actually age better.

In a study conducted by the *British Journal for Sports Medicine,* it was discovered that even those who were just beginning a regular exercise routine over the age of sixty became categorized as healthy agers by the time the four-year study ended. The benefits of regular exercise for older adults is monumental.

Older adults who get regular exercise are not only healthier physically, but also mentally, cognitively, and emotionally. Occurrences of dementia and Alzheimer's are less frequent in more active adults. Another wonderful benefit of exercise? Not having to worry about numerous medications!

I would like to give you a friendly word of encouragement. Even though exercise at any age is beneficial, don't wait until you're old and beginning to feel the effects of your poor choices before you make healthier ones. Exercise and movement are valuable at any age!

The reason I exercise is for the quality of life I enjoy.
KENNETH H. COOPER

HOW EXERCISE CAN HELP YOUR BRAIN

As I mentioned before, one of the many benefits of regular exercise is increased cognition and memory. Those who exercise more tend to be more alert and find it easier to concentrate. Also, movement prevents harmful toxins from building up in your brain, by supplying more oxygen.

Studies have shown that exercise in your youth can affect your cognition and focus in middle age. Knowing this, it's a good idea to lead a healthy and active lifestyle during all phases in life!

PHYSICAL ACTIVITY AND
PAIN RELIEF

Have you ever found when you have a pulled muscle or other muscular ailment that movement actually helps it to feel better? Being active and pursuing regular exercise can actually help you to limit your pain. By gaining flexibility in your joints and moving your muscles, you can also help prevent injury. Older adults who are more active experience less chronic pain and fewer health issues.

Barbara, a retired psychotherapist, was very active for someone in her seventies and enjoyed traveling. Unfortunately, on her last trip to India she fell and ended up in the hospital with a broken hip. It had taken her months to recover. Her biggest problem was that as she began to age, she began to experience more difficulty with balance. And she is not alone.

Each year 2.5 million older people are treated for fall injuries. Over 700,000 patients a year are hospitalized because of a fall injury. Falls are the most common cause of traumatic brain injury and broken hips. Many of those falls are caused by difficulties with walking and balance. You might have balance issues yourself or wonder what you can do to improve your balance. This is where t'ai chi, yoga, and qigong come in.

To enjoy the glow of good health, you must exercise.

GENE TUNNEY

THE BENEFITS OF T'AI CHI,
YOGA, AND QIGONG

Knowing that exercise and mobility play a huge role in physical and mental health as we age, it makes sense to look at some forms of movement that can help you to find the maximum benefits of exercise. The practices of t'ai chi, yoga, and qigong have been proven to provide more energy than you put into them. That's good news, since most people find that their busy lifestyles drain them of the energy necessary to obtain regular exercise.

Not only do these forms of exercise rejuvenate our bodies, but they also strengthen our minds and balance. They are time proven, being practiced for thousands of years in Eastern cultures.

When I traveled to China, I was amazed at how many elderly people were in a park doing t'ai chi. In San Francisco and in Chinatown, it was the same thing. Did these elderly people know something that we don't?

T'ai Chi

T'ai chi is practiced alongside ancient Chinese medicine to help promote healing and health. Similar in many ways to yoga, t'ai chi focuses on movement and being in tune with your body. By being cognizant of your body and its motions, it is believed that you can promote your own healing, balance, and prolonged health.

The practice of t'ai chi is part of traditional Chinese medicine. It is thought that focusing your energy can promote healing and overall health. Rather than focusing on the one ailing part, t'ai chi focuses on the entire body and its energy flow.

While modern exercise focuses on rapid movement, t'ai chi does just the opposite. The constant but slow dancelike movements promote balance and focus. With the slow and deliberate movements associated with t'ai chi, even those who are physically limited can get ample exercise and enjoy the benefits of physical activity.

Studies have shown that t'ai chi helps to strengthen your central nervous system, aiding in better mobility and range of motion. Those who are older or are limited in their movements or are experiencing balance issues can greatly benefit from this aspect of the exercise.

Link between T'ai Chi and Increased Brain Function

T'ai chi has amazing effects when it comes to cognition and brain function. Those who practiced it on a regular basis were less forgetful, more alert, and better able to follow conversations. Regular movement and exercise helps blood flow to the brain, aiding in higher levels of cognition and alertness.

Healing Chronic Health Problems

As people age, arthritis and other joint and muscle problems tend to surface. The great thing about t'ai chi is that it can be used by people who suffer from arthritis and mobility issues. Due to its low impact and slow movements, people who suffer with chronic pain have found it beneficial to their conditions as well.

While there is still much research being conducted concerning t'ai chi, it may be the prescription of the future. Those with chronic illnesses such as cancer have benefited healthwise from the practice of t'ai chi.

Links to Stem-Cell Research

While researching the benefits of t'ai chi, it has been discovered that the practice actually aids in the formation of stem cells. Those who practiced t'ai chi saw an increase in their blood stem cells, which in turn aids in regeneration.

Yoga

As we age we become more inflexible in body and mind. For this reason, it is important to maintain our flexibility. Two of the most common health issues that arise from inflexibility are arthritis and chronic pain.

Back pain is one of the most common medical problems affecting eight out of ten people at some point in their lives. Lower back pain affects about 80 percent of people and 20 to 30 percent are recurrent. There are a large number of Americans who, after trying many standard treatments, are still left with serious back pain. My neighbor is one of those people. He already had back surgery once, but his back is still a problem. I have found that the best way to treat back pain, in fact any kind of physical pain including arthritis, is through prevention. Yoga is one of the best preventive ways to do this. My yoga teacher would always say, "You're as young as your spine."

The practice of yoga has become more prevalent in the United States in the last few decades. You can hardly drive a block in California without seeing a yoga studio. This form of physical and mental exercise focuses on the link between your mind and body. During the poses, or *asanas,* you are focused on your body and its movement, your breathing, and your muscles.

Yoga has been proven to help with flexibility and mobility, as well as weight loss and the prevention of mental health problems. By having a relaxed and focused mind, those who practice yoga are less stressed out and better able to cope with life.

Benefits of Yoga

Ancient yoga focused on the mind and body connection, but modern yoga adds physical movement into the mix with stretches and stances. By adding the physical aspects of yoga, those who practice yoga have found that they are living a healthier and longer life.

Many seek yoga because of its many benefits. Not only is yoga helpful in calming your mind and relaxing your body, but it also helps lower blood pressure, ease feelings of stress and anxiety, and promote movement and muscle control. The focus part of yoga helps to sharpen your focus and promotes higher levels of cognition.

Not only is it good for the body, it's good for the mind and mood. Studies have found that the practice of yoga can reduce the feelings of anxiety, depression, and other mood disorders.

Yoga has also been shown to aid in weight loss by improving leptin sensitivity. Leptin is a hormone that regulates your energy levels based upon movement. Those who practiced yoga were found to have a higher leptin sensitivity, helping them to lose weight and feel healthier.

I have been practicing yoga for forty-two years and have observed people my age who haven't done yoga. Their range of motion is extremely limited. They are not at ease in their body and suffer from arthritis, and many aches and pains that they incorrectly attribute to aging. They look older than their years, and their posture is beginning to stoop. Regularly practicing yoga will keep you flexible in body and mind and allow your body to repair itself more rapidly and create an upright and flexible spine.

Qigong

I believe Qigong can be one of the best things one can do as one ages to help regenerate the body by eliminating energy blockages both mentally and physically, thereby allowing the free flow of chi, which I have come to believe is the real secret behind vitality and vibrant health.

What Is Qigong?

As mentioned earlier, qigong isn't necessarily focused on motion like yoga, as much as it's focused on the energy that flows through your body. Qigong is a practice that goes alongside t'ai chi, combining motion and focusing on energy flow.

Essentially, qigong is focused on using inner energy for healing. Working together with traditional Chinese medicine, it is believed that using your inner forces can aid in healing and longevity. In Chinese hospitals, in addition to acupuncturists, there are qigong healers.

Qigong and Chinese Medicine

Traditional Chinese medicine vastly differs from Western medicine. In our world, we are used to fixing a certain part if it's ailing, or in masking the pain, in other words treating symptomatically. In Chinese medicine, the body is regarded as a whole, with an energy flow that determines the body's overall health. If you find that you are feeling ill, it is due to a blockage in energy, and that blockage must be removed in order to heal.

Chinese medicine focuses more on the overall picture rather than individual parts, and on healing rather than managing pain. Qigong aids this practice in helping the body self-heal by breaking down the energy blockages that the body is experiencing. This is accomplished through meditation and mantras, focusing on bringing positive energy throughout the body.

Qigong health practice is based on gentle movements, meditation, and breathing, which, like acupuncture, is believed to help the chi, or energy, move more easily through your body and therefore has a wide range of benefits including improving balance, lowering blood pressure, and even easing depression.

Benefits of Qigong

While it may seem strange for you to think of your body as having an energy that promotes health, qigong has had many success stories. The benefits of practicing qigong consist of, but are not limited to:

- Less need for medications
- A natural way to promote health and well-being

- Avoiding unnecessary medical care and procedures
- Loosening tight muscles and aiding in gaining strength—the Chinese think of muscular strength as being inappropriate, so they focus on relaxation rather than strength training
- Strengthening your organs—qigong provides strength and balance for your internal organs, for a sense of overall well-being
- Improving cardiovascular health
- Strengthening your nerves
- Can be used for all activity levels
- Helping prevent muscle and joint injury
- Aiding in lessening recovery times
- Easing stress and aiding in mood and sleep
- Increasing efficiency of your metabolism
- Benefiting those with limited mobility and movement

Qigong has many wonderful health benefits that would fit into any lifestyle. Just because you may not be physically able to exercise, focusing your body's energy can help aid in your health and healing.

Qigong and Healing

It is said that by performing qigong regularly, you will look and feel better. Even for those who have limited mobility, the act of positivity derived from this practice makes them feel healthier and more energetic.

MOVEMENT AND ITS BENEFITS

It's no secret that we can benefit from regular exercise. Studies have shown time and again that regular exercise leads to a healthier life. However, we tend to just look at the studies and keep on doing what we have done before. Have you ever thought of the fact that what you do today will somehow affect your future? You may not think that sitting in front of the television today will affect your health, but being sedentary on a regular basis will have a negative impact on your health over time.

Let's take a look at some of the benefits that you can reap from having regular movement and exercise in your life.

Having a healthy, flexible body and feeling good are just the obvious benefits of exercise. There are many more benefits to regular exercise and movement than just being comfortable in your body and feeling healthy. Studies have shown that increased movement and exercise has direct links to increased brain function. The more you move, the more alert you can be, the better you can think and continue to concentrate even as you age.

Walking

One of the most popular and easiest ways to exercise is walking. A study done by Dr. Mercola found that walking just twenty minutes a day showed a significant increase in brain function, as well as limiting the tendency to succumb to illness. Another research study done by John J. Ratey indicates that exercise can protect your brain and its function by:

- Increasing blood flow to the brain
- Increasing the production of nerve-protecting compounds
- Aiding in the development and protection of neurons
- Cleansing your brain of the damaging protein, amyloid beta, linked to Alzheimer's disease

With so many benefits, don't you want to get your body into motion in order to protect your brain?

Daily Walking

Yes, we all walk and do it without a thought. When we talk about daily walking here, we are talking about walking consistently for a period of time without stopping. Just walking for twenty minutes a day can increase your life by seven years and help in aging more gracefully! Not only do you get physical activity, but you also get exposed to the sun, which provides vitamin D. You can even walk barefoot and enjoy the feel of the ground beneath your feet! The electrons in the soil can be beneficial to your health as well.

Walking Can Reduce Your Risk of Chronic Illness

Along with other types of movement, walking on a regular basis can reduce your risk of chronic illness. Those who walked on a regular basis showed less tendency to have heart disease, cancer, osteoporosis, and other chronic health problems. Just by making an effort to get out and enjoy the beautiful outdoors, you are helping yourself to live longer and feel healthier!

The Benefits of Dancing

Looking at movement and motion, we also need to look at the benefits of dancing for older adults. In studies, it has been found that the elderly people who danced on a regular basis experienced less hip and knee pain and increased flexibility. Those in the study found that they experienced less stiffness and could move more quickly. This can really benefit older adults when they wish to stay independent for as long as possible.

I enjoy line dancing and belly dancing because in addition to its physical benefits, it's really fun!

POINTS TO REMEMBER

Increasing your movement can have numerous positive effects on your health and aging. In particular, the practices of t'ai chi, yoga, and qigong have been practiced for thousands of years in Eastern cultures. Having a mind and body connection can help you to be more aware of your body's needs and take better care of your health. These low-impact exercises not only help with your body's flexibility, but they also make you aware of your body in ways that you never thought of before.

Being more aware of your body and exercising can help your body to age better and it can help to protect your brain against disease. Those who get regular movement, including walking and dancing, have better memory and are more aware of what is going on around them. This is especially important for those who are entering their golden years, as memory tends to fade and older adults develop Alzheimer's and dementia more frequently.

Healthy aging and brain protection should start at any stage of your life. Don't worry if you haven't had the best of habits up until this point. Start today and continue for the rest of your life. Knowing that studies have proven that movement can help you age better and healthier, why don't we want to get the ball rolling now?

I encourage you to take the time to get regular movement and exercise on a daily basis. Look for opportunities to be active. Since what you do today will affect your health and well-being in the future, why not set yourself up for a healthy and active second half?

REFERENCES FOR CHAPTER 18

BBC News. "Tai Chi 'Could Be Prescribed' for Illnesses." September 18, 2015. www.bbc.co.uk/news/health-34279190 (accessed May 6, 2017).

Bond, Annie B. "The Twelve Benefits of Qigong." *Care2,* May 2, 2005. www.care2 .com/greenliving/the-twelve-benefits-of-qigong.html (accessed May 6, 2017).

Cardiff University. "35 Year Study Finds Exercise Reduces Risk of Dementia." *Science Daily,* December 9, 2013. www.sciencedaily.com/releases/2013 /12/131209181059.htm (accessed May 6, 2017).

Collins, Nick. "Exercise in Sixties Boosts Healthy Ageing." *Telegraph,* November 26, 2013. www.telegraph.co.uk/news/health/elder/10473312/Exercise-in -sixties-boosts-healthy-ageing.html (accessed May 6, 2017).

———. "Tai Chi and Yoga Could Prevent Fall Injuries in Elderly." *Telegraph,* October 29, 2013. www.telegraph.co.uk/news/health/elder/10411825 /Tai-Chi-and-yoga-could-prevent-fall-injuries-in-elderly.html (accessed May 6, 2017).

Druda, Angelo. "Secrets of Longevity Yoga." *Natural News,* September 9, 2013. www.naturalnews.com/041967_longevity_yoga_secrets_rejuvenation.html (accessed May 6, 2017).

Eliaz, Isaac. "Why Yoga, Tai Chi, and Qi Gong Aren't Like Other Workouts." *MindBodyGreen,* July 10, 2012. www.mindbodygreen.com/0-5423/Why -Yoga-Tai-Chi-and-Qi-Gong-Arent-Like-Other-Workouts.html (accessed May 6, 2017).

EnergyArts. "Qigong Benefits." www.energyarts.com/qigong-benefits (accessed May 6, 2017).

Louis, P. F. "Only 20 Minutes of Yoga Instantly Stimulates the Brain: Study." *Natural News,* June 14, 2013. www.naturalnews.com/040763_yoga_brain _stimulation_mind-body_medicine.html (accessed May 6, 2017).

———. "Yoga Is a 'Life Changing' Practice That Reduces Bipolar Symptoms, Anxiety, Depression, and More." *Natural News,* October 9, 2014. www .naturalnews.com/047187_yoga_bipolar_mental_health.html (accessed May 6, 2017).

Mercola, Joseph. "Does Exercise Change Your Brain?" *Mercola,* September 18, 2015. http://fitness.mercola.com/sites/fitness/archive/2015/09/18/exercise -brain-health.aspx (accessed May 6, 2017).

———. "New Study: Daily Walk Can Add 7 Years to Your Life." *Mercola,* September 11, 2015. http://fitness.mercola.com/sites/fitness/archive/2015/09 /11/daily-walk-benefits.aspx (accessed May 6, 2017).

———. "Strengthening Your Body Strengthens Your Mind." *Mercola,* November 27, 2015. http://fitness.mercola.com/sites/fitness/archive/2015/11/27/strength -training-brain-health.aspx (accessed May 6, 2017).

———. "Tai Chi and Other Low-Impact Exercises May Be Ideal for Elderly People with Chronic Health Problems." *Mercola,* October 9, 2015. http:// fitness.mercola.com/sites/fitness/archive/2015/10/09/tai-chi-benefits.aspx (accessed May 6, 2017).

Nemour, Stacey. "Qigong: Unleash Incredible Healing Powers." *HuffPost,* July 21, 2010. www.huffingtonpost.com/stacey-nemour/qigong-unleash -incredible_b_651561.html (accessed May 6, 2017).

Preidt, Robert. "Dance Away That Arthritis Pain." *Everyday Health,* June 30, 2014. www.everydayhealth.com/news/dance-away-that-arthritis-pain (accessed May 6, 2017).

Ragnar, Peter. "Does Qi Gong Really Work?" *Longevity Sage,* www.longevitysage .com/does-qigong-really-work/ (accessed May 6, 2017).

Tong, Gary. "Qi Gong." *A Touch of Chi,* April 13, 2013. www.atouchofchi.com /qigong (accessed May 6, 2017).

University of Eastern Finland. "Physical Activity Is Beneficial for Late-Life Cognition." *Science Daily,* April 9, 2014. www.sciencedaily.com /releases/2014/04/140409094045.htm (accessed May 6, 2017).

WorldHealth.net. "Tai Chi Enhances Stem Cells." June 30, 2014. www .worldhealth.net/news/tai-chi-enhances-stem-cells/ (accessed May 6, 2017).

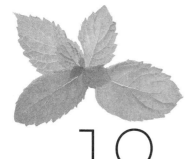

19

ALL THE RESOURCES YOU NEED ARE AT YOUR FINGERTIPS

If you think the pursuit of good health is expensive and time consuming, try illness.

Lee Swanson (Swanson Health Products)

It's time to think about the pursuit of good health. What is interesting about the above quote is the word *pursuit*. The definition of *pursuit* is, "the action of following or pursuing something, an effort to secure or attain, a quest."

In other words, one cannot be passive about good health but must actively engage in activities that bring or promote it.

Cheers to people who do their own research. In this age of information, ignorance is a choice and when it comes to your health, ignorance is not bliss. Ignorance is a virtual life sentence to unnecessary pain and discomfort.

KNOWLEDGE IS POWER

Most people don't realize it, but when armed with the right knowledge and natural therapies, they are more capable of healing their bodies than they ever imagined.

DR. JULIAN WHITAKER

At the present time the U.S. Health System almost entirely ignores nutrition in favor of pharmacology.

DR. WALTER WILLET, HARVARD SCHOOL
OF PUBLIC HEALTH

We had not been back from Florida to visit our New York friends in three years. I was amazed to discover how their health had seriously deteriorated in so short a time. Most were in their seventies and eighties. The once thriving and lively individuals had succumbed to chronic disease and illness, while my husband and I were still fit and healthy.

They almost all, without exception, had serious chronic health issues and were on multiple prescription medications. The illnesses ranged from heart problems to dementia, cancer, Parkinson's, severe arthritis, needing hip or knee replacements, and more. In fact, we were supposed to meet with a couple when we got a call that the husband was in the hospital having a stent put in. One friend had five stents. Another friend had passed away with heart disease.

These are people who are extremely busy. I began to think about time and how you spend your time. I also began to think about aging and how you spend the last third of your life, and how much the quality of your life is determined by lifestyle choices. The prevailing mode of thinking became quite clear: You live your life, and when you're sick you go to the doctor and he gives you a prescription. The priority was enjoying your life even if that meant drinking in excess, eating very late at night, or even eating extremely unhealthy foods. The underlying assumption is I've earned this, and I can do what I want.

There is a big difference between simply becoming old, and aging consciously, with intent.

People need to make the decision that they want to actively pursue good health and wellness, because without health you really have nothing. No matter how much money or power you have, you can't live your life freely. Living freely means without pain and suffering. You can't sit around and play cards all day, eat late at night, and drink in excess, and expect to reap the benefits of good health. A sedentary lifestyle will bring a sedentary future. Life is about adventure and freedom. If you are encumbered by poor health, you have no freedom to enjoy the pleasures that you have earned or have been given.

> **Every time you eat or drink, you are either feeding disease or fighting it.**

I would like to share a story with you that I believe nicely illustrates this thought process. As I grow older, I still look back to this time in my life and compare it to how people choose to age.

When I was a child growing up in Brooklyn, New York, my father would take my sister, brother, and me to Coney Island on the weekends. He would give us each a handful of pennies to spend as we wished on rides, food, and arcade machines. I was very careful about how I spent my pennies. I wanted to get the most bang for my buck. I wanted to have fun, but I also wanted the fun to last for as long as possible.

Life is like that too. We are given a handful of years and need to make the decision about how to spend it. Some people choose to squander their years, others choose to spend wisely. Ask yourself this question: Is what you're doing pursuing life or death, health or disease, happiness or misery?

> *Two roads diverged in a wood, and I . . . I took the one less traveled by, and that has made all the difference.*
>
> ROBERT FROST

THE NEW PARADIGM OF HEALTH

I have time on my mind today and how we use it. People love telling everyone else how busy they are. As if the mere fact of being busy had its own intrinsic value. However, being busy to fill your days is not the end all.

Far more valuable is the idea that at the end of the day, you have achieved something constructive.

Today more than at any other time in history we have the power to reinvent ourselves and restructure our lives in a new way, to allow new ideas to come into our lives, to rethink old ways, to break old patterns, and to gift ourselves with more free time.

What my friends were not yet aware of is that the old paradigm of medicine is rapidly dying. People are becoming aware of the limitations of modern medicine, which basically is centered on controlling symptoms but not really curing the disease itself. They fail to understand that taking responsibility for our health is not an option, it's a necessity. Society has made frailty and old-age ailments seem like they are something normal and to be expected. They are not. Don't allow the current paradigm to dictate how you age and progress through life.

Why can't we all be centenarians? Think about that for a while. As we begin to take care of our entire health, life expectancies will grow longer, making it possible to live a longer and healthier life. Don't set yourself back based upon what is considered normal. Use your body's regenerative qualities to allow you to live longer and feel better!

A new paradigm of medicine is slowly emerging, much like new life springing from the ashes after a fire. This new paradigm focuses on the regenerative capacities of the body through a specific plan encompassing diet, supplementation, natural hormones, adaptogens, and energy medicine.

This paradigm is coupled with the rapidly emerging field of regenerative medicine that incorporates 3-D printing of organs, stem cells, growing new body parts, and gene manipulation. This combination has the potential to create real health, not just symptom suppression.

My book provides readers with the information they need to enhance the body's capacity for regeneration. This concept has largely been ignored by Western medicine, but is deeply entrenched in many other types of medicines such as traditional Chinese medicine; energy medicine; herbal, traditional, and native medicine. Additionally, we need to understand that healing needs to occur on all levels, not just at the level of the physical symptoms. Healing needs to occur in the body, mind, and spirit. This will be part of this new paradigm and what it sets out to achieve.

The purpose of *The Miracle of Regenerative Medicine* is to give readers the necessary tools and resources so they can participate in their own wellness. With all the information that I have thrown in your direction, I want you to understand this: healing is all about our entire being, not just feeling good physically. That is just a small piece of the overall puzzle.

In this paradigm, aging people will begin to realize that they don't need to delegate their health to an "expert." People will begin to realize that they are ultimately responsible for their individual health. They will come to realize that an "ounce of prevention is worth a pound of cure." People will become more in touch with their own true nature and trust their intuition as opposed to an outside authority. That doesn't mean not going to a health care professional. Rather it is important to get a diagnosis, and once that is done, decisions need to be made about how they want to handle what's wrong with them.

This emerging paradigm requires a new way of navigating. Those who have become aware of the incoming energy shift will likely notice that approaches that worked in the past now fall flat or actually backfire. Habits like pushing away uncomfortable feelings, distracting ourselves with low-vibrational entertainment and food, manipulating and trying to control others, and concealing our flaws with fancy adornments no longer yield satisfying results.

Sure we can still employ these old methods, but as many have discovered, the more awake we are, the less effective and ultimately the less rewarding these strategies will be. We can sit by and live the old way as long as we want, but we will ultimately fail at making ourselves feel good under the old paradigm.

The new paradigm will provide many treatment options other than prescription drugs, which are often expensive and produce a multitude of side effects. We live in an age of information, and people who are in touch with their bodies and mind can and will objectively make an assessment and avail themselves of many options. Some of these options we have discussed in this book.

They may go to an alternative/complementary physician, a naturopathic physician, an acupuncturist, or a homeopath. These practices will treat with natural medicine. Becoming more proactive about prevention, engaging in energy enhancing activities like qigong, t'ai chi, and yoga are just a few ways that people can experience total wellness.

People are already beginning to realize the role of the mind in illness and taking up meditation. They might begin a gratitude practice or prayer. They will come to appreciate and live every day of their lives knowing that time is the most precious commodity. They will begin to maximize their time by engaging in life-enhancing activities rather than life-destroying habits. They will become gentler with themselves, allowing them to be gentler with others as well. They will begin to socialize with others and have healthy, supportive relationships.

While you are walking away from this book with a wealth of new knowledge, I have found that I too have learned many valuable lessons in my research. What I learned in the last ten years of researching this book includes:

- The best diet is a whole-foods, plant-based diet with roots in tradition, which means time-proven foods (not necessarily a vegetarian diet).
- The concept of inflammation is the root cause of practically every disease.
- Your gut microbiome (the bacteria that reside in your intestines) is a vital part of your health and fermented foods keep it that way, as does fiber. Your gut microbiome changes after each meal. It controls not only mood, but immunity and inflammation.
- Your thoughts manifest your reality. You are what you think. Every cell in your body has "cellular intelligence" and will respond to your thoughts.
- Exercise is not optional as you age, but a requirement. Use it or lose it.
- You're as young as your spine. Keep your body and mind flexible.
- Change your thoughts, change your life; an attitude of gratitude makes all the difference between a positive and negative mind-set.
- We are much more than body, tissue, and bones, but are actually energetic beings. If you keep your energy flowing through your body, without obstructions, you can not only create health but heal body, mind, and spirit.
- Your body's ability to heal is greater than they have ever led you to believe.

- When it comes to your health, ignorance is not bliss.
- Many chronic and debilitating illnesses that we associate with age can actually be prevented.
- You need to become not only informed but proactive about your health.
- Suppression of symptoms is not a cure. Taking away pain is not healing.
- You are responsible for your health and well-being, not your doctor.
- There are many supplements that can assist and support your health.
- Aging is part of life, but looking and feeling old and becoming frail are optional.
- Your genes are not your destiny.

Release fear and all that it prevents you from doing. Instead cultivate your intuition and combine it with this newly discovered knowledge and you will no longer be dependent on any medication, any doctor, or even any system. You'll be in your power. This is the new medicine. It's a revolutionary paradigm that makes the old one obsolete.

KELLY BROGAN, M.D.

POINTS TO REMEMBER

Just because you are growing old, doesn't mean that you must have multiple diseases and suffer from poor health. Learning how the body works and how you can use its regenerative properties to allow for optimal health will help our society shift to a new paradigm. In this new paradigm, old age doesn't mean ill health. It means being healthy and enjoying life.

I have seen too many people allow disease and age to rob them of the enjoyment life has to offer. Now is the time to make these changes in your life and allow yourself the reward of living a healthy and happy existence.

I have learned tons from researching and writing this book. However, the one thing that will always stick with me is that my health is my choice. I am in control of how I age and how I feel. With that knowledge, I choose to embrace my overall health.

Are you ready to enjoy your life? If so, I encourage you to shift your thought process of what aging tends to encompass and use your body's natural abilities to heal and regenerate. Life offers you many chances to make these changes. Don't allow the common misconception that age means frailty to control your life.

Take the time and figure out what you want from your life and health. Then use those goals to make changes to your lifestyle. Changing your mind-set is the first step in pursuing a long and healthy life.

🖋

Now I understand what you tried to say . . . and how you tried to set them free. They would not listen, they did not know how. Perhaps they'll listen now.

DON MCLEAN, "STARRY STARRY NIGHT"

RESOURCES
FOR WELLNESS

This book covered many different ideas for healthy living and wellness through natural medicine and alternative therapies. I used multiple resources to research these topics. These institutes and individuals are the leaders in their respective fields and so I recommend that you go through the resources mentioned in this section and check out the ones you are interested in or that might be beneficial to you.

ALTERNATIVE/COMPLEMENTARY
HEALTH CARE

Whitaker Wellness Institute
www.whitakerwellness.com
The Whitaker Wellness Institute in Newport Beach, California, was opened in 1979 by Julian Whitaker, M.D., to provide natural medicine, nutritional and lifestyle advice, and alternative therapies under one roof for those who had been let down by conventional medicine. Dr. Whitaker has authored thirteen books on healthy living, writes a monthly newsletter, Health & Healing, that has millions of subscribers, and has founded the Freedom of Health Foundation, a nonprofit that works on educating people about natural and alternative therapies.

Life Extension Foundation
www.lifeextensionfoundation.org

Life Extension Foundation is a nonprofit institute founded in 1980 to fund scientific research into areas of extending human life-span, anti-aging research, and fighting diseases such as cancer, stroke, heart disease, and Alzheimer's.

Tahoma Clinic
www.tahomaclinic.com

Dr. Jonathan V. Wright, a world-leading pioneer in natural medicine, started the Tahoma Clinic in 1973 to provide evidence-based natural treatments to patients. The clinics are located in Tukwila and North Seattle, Washington.

South California Center for Anti-Aging
www.socalbhrt.com

South California Center for Anti-Aging in Torrance, California, is the clinic of Judy Goldstein, M.D., an anti-aging and weight loss expert. She has been practicing wellness medicine since 2001 and has been a member of the American Academy of Anti-aging and Regenerative Medicine since 2005.

Health Integration Center
www.healthintegrationcenter.net

The Health Integration Center was founded in 1978 by David Y. Wong, M.D., to provide an integrated approach to wellness that included both conventional medicine and evidence-based natural medicine. The Torrance, California based clinic focuses on healing the mind, body, and spirit.

National Center for Complementary and Integrative Health
www.nccih.nih.gov

CAM (Complementary and Alternative Medical Professionals) is a term that covers all the doctors and physicians that offer natural and alternative therapies different from the conventional medicine. The National Center for Complementary and Integrative Health is a government organization that will give you all the information you need before selecting a CAM professional.

American Association of Naturopathic Physicians (AANP)
www.naturopathic.org
AANP, founded in 1985, is the premier association for naturopathic doctors and physicians in the United States. It is a good place to find an accredited naturopathic doctor near you and learn about the latest developments in naturopathic medicine.

American Naturopathic Medical Association (ANMA)
www.anma.org
ANMA, founded in 1981, is the oldest and largest association of naturopathic doctors in the United States. It is a nonprofit organization that works on education, exploration of naturopathic medicine, and fighting legislation that would hinder the growth of naturopathic medicine.

WHERE TO GET . . .

PRP Therapy

You can get PRP therapy in most integrated or alternative clinics. Doctors practicing sports medicine are experienced with PRP and most of them offer it to other patients as well.

Stem Cells

PlacidWay U.S. Medical Tourism (www.placidway.com) in Denver helps patients find the best location for stem-cell therapy in the United States and around the world.

Other leading centers for stem-cell research are:

New York Stem Cell Treatment Center (www.nystemcellcenter.com)

Stem Genex Medical Group (www.stemgenex.com)

Aspen Institute for Anti-aging & Regenerative Medicine (http://aspen-regenerativemedicine.com/)

Invictus Healthcare System, Tulsa (www.invictushealthcaresystem.com)

Regenerex (www.regenerex.com)

Regenerative Medicine Foundation (www.regmedfoundation.org)

Wake Forest Institute for Regenerative Medicine (www.wakehealth.edu/WFIRM/)

International Society for Stem Cell Research (www.isscr.org)

Centre for Regenerative Medicine (www.crm.ed.ac.uk)

Mayo Clinic Transplant Center (www.mayoclinic.org/departments
-centers/transplant-center/regenerative-medicine-consultation
-service/gnc-20203917)

University of Miami, Miller School of Medicine, Interdisciplinary
Stem Cell Institute (www.isci.med.miami.edu)

UC Davis Stem Cell Program (www.ucdmc.ucdavis.edu/
stemcellresearch/)

Qigong

International College of Medical Qigong (www.medicalqigong.org),
founded by Dr. Bernard Shannon, offers courses in qigong and has a clinical directory for clinics opened by their graduates.

The Qigong Research and Practice Center (www.qigonghealing.com)
provides educational courses as well as healing and consultation.

Chiyan Wang of Taoist Light Qigong (www.taoistlightqigong.com) in
Santa Barbara, California, teaches Taoist Light qigong, which has been
passed through a long lineage of teachers at the Lao Guan Tai Temple in
China going all the way back to Lao Tzu himself.

If you want to read books about Qigong, the **International Institute of
Medical Qigong Publishing House, Inc.** (www.qigongmedicine.com) is
the place to start.

Hyperbaric Oxygen Treatment

Hyperbaric Link (www.hyperbariclink.com) has a directory of all the
treatment centers in the United States. Most conventional hospitals now
offer hyperbaric oxygen therapy.

Mayo Clinic (www.mayoclinic.org) has one of the largest hyperbaric oxygen therapy chambers in the United States.

Whitaker Wellness Center Institute (www.whitakerwellness.com) also
offers hyperbaric oxygen therapy.

Yoga

You can find a yoga studio with ease in most big cities. This page: www
.gyanunlimited.com/health/list-of-top-10-yoga-studios-of-united-states-of
-america-usa, offers a list of the top yoga studios in the biggest cities of the
United States. There are also tons of online resources, such as websites, books,
videos, and online courses, for you to learn yoga from the comfort of your home.

Medical Cannabis

Medical Cannabis is legal in twenty-eight states in the United States.
Link to the list: (http://medicalmarijuana.procon.org/view.resource.
php?resourceID=000881).

CannaCraft (www.cannacraft.com) is the premium medical cannabis pro-
ducer in California. They produce strain-specific cannabis oil, CBD medicines, artisanal cannabis chocolates, and cannabis-infused lotions and balms.

Medicinal Marijuana Association (www.medicinalmarijuanaassociation
.com) is a good place to find all the information you need about medical
marijuana.

T'ai Chi

Supreme Chi Living (www.americantaichi.net) and Tai Chi Foundation
(www.taichifoundation.org) are two great sites to find information about
t'ai chi and also locate a class near you. Just like yoga, you can also use
online resources to learn more about it on your own.

Acupuncture

Acupuncture has become very popular in the United States and you can
find an acupuncturist in alternative clinics and even some conventional
hospitals. This page of the **Acupuncture Now Foundation** can help you
locate a qualified acupuncturist in your area:
(https://acupuncturenowfoundation.org/find-qualified-acupuncturist-usa).

Homeopathy

The National Center for Homeopathy (NCH) (www.homeopathycenter
.org), the **North American Society for Homeopaths** (NASH) (www

.homeopathy.org), and the **American Institute of Homeopathy** (www
.homeopathyusa.org) are great resources to find out more about homeopathy
and also to find licensed homeopathic doctors and clinics in your area.

Homeopathic Educational Services (www.homeopathic.com) is a good
place to learn about homeopathy.

WHERE TO BUY VITAMINS, SUPPLEMENTS, AND HOMEOPATHIC MEDICINE

Whole Foods stores carry a large variety of vitamins, supplements, and
even homeopathic medicines.

Boiron is a world leader in homeopathic medicine and many stores such as
Whole Foods, Target, Walmart, Walgreens, and CVS Pharmacy carry their
range of medicines. You can also buy their medicines online and through
mail-order services.

Hyland's is another reputable manufacturer of homeopathic medicine
and you can use the store locator on their website to find a store near you:
(www.hylands.com/product-locator#search/local/default).

Heel is a pioneer pharmaceutical company that manufactures medicines
from all-natural ingredients.

Swanson Health Products (www.swansonvitamins.com) provides all
kinds of natural supplements, herbal medicines, vitamins, and homeopathic remedies.

Mushroom Wisdom (www.mushroomwisdom.com) specializes in mushroom supplements. Their supplements are available in over a thousand
stores in the United States and they have fourteen international distribut-
ers. You can locate the store near you on their website.

Emerson Ecologics (www.emersonecologics.com) is a one-stop online
shop for all kinds of natural medicine, supplements, skin care products,
homeopathic medicine, and the like.

Life Extension (www.lifeextension.com) is a good place to buy vitamins,
minerals, supplements, and natural skin care products.

Willner Chemists (www.willner.com) on Park Ave, in New York City, is a great place to buy nutritional supplements. They've been around since 1911 and today are the top-rated nutritional pharmacy in the country. You can also buy their supplements online through their website.

Dr. Whitaker (www.drwhitaker.com), the founder of the Whitaker Wellness Institute, also has an online store where you can by vitamins and other supplements.

The Bach Center is a good source of information about Bach Flower remedies.

BOOKS WORTH READING

Female and Forgetful by Elisa Lottor

Vibrational Medicine by Richard Gerber, M.D.

The Bach Flower Remedies by Edward Bach, M.D., and F. J. Wheeler, M.D.

The Complete Homeopathy Handbook: Safe and Effective Ways to Treat Fevers, Coughs, Colds and Sore Throats, Childhood Ailments, Food Poisoning, Flu, and a Wide Range of Everyday Complaints by Miranda Castro

The Science of Homeopathy by George Vithoulkas

The Encyclopedia of Natural Medicine by Michael T. Murray

Alternative Medicine: The Definitive Guide by Burton Goldberg and John W. Anderson

The Medical Cannabis Guidebook: The Definitive Guide to Using and Growing Medicinal Marijuana by Jeff Ditchfield and Mel Thomas

Light on Yoga: Yoga Dipika by B. K. S. Iyengar, with foreword by Yehudi Menuhin

The Complete Illustrated Book of Yoga by Swami Vishnu Devananda

The Way of Qigong: The Art and Science of Chinese Energy Healing by Ken Cohen

Lao Tzu: Tao Te Ching by Ursula K. Le Guin

T'ai Chi Ch'uan: Technique of Power by H. H. Lui and Tem Horwitz

Tao Te Ching by Stephen Mitchell

INDEX